KW-053-969

BRITISH MEDICAL BULLETIN — Volume 52 Number 1 January 1996

Tobacco and health

Scientific Editors

Sir Richard Doll and Sir John Crofton

Acknowledgements

The committee that planned this number of the *British Medical Bulletin* was chaired by Professor Sir Richard Doll and also included Professor Sir John Crofton, Mr David Pollock, Professor Michael A H Russell and Professor Nicholas J Wald.

The British Council and Royal Society of Medicine Press are most grateful to them for their help and advice, and particularly to Professors Doll and Crofton for their work as Scientific Editors.

Preface

Tobacco smoking is now generally accepted as the most important cause of premature death, and of much chronic ill health, in most industrialised countries. In recent years, the habit has been increasing in many developing countries, fostered by ruthless marketing by the multinational tobacco companies. Sadly, in these countries, this will add a further burden of smoking-related disease to their already heavy burdens of communicable disease and malnutrition and to the disease for which, in some of them, other and traditional forms of tobacco use, such as chewing, have long been responsible. Commercial pressures are also increasing tobacco smoking in many Eastern European countries, threatening to worsen a health record that is already causing much international concern.

In consequence of these trends, The British Council thought it appropriate to devote a special issue of the *British Medical Bulletin* to tobacco smoking. The aim has been to produce summaries of the effects of smoking both on those who smoke and on those who are exposed involuntarily to smoke in the environment, to review the strategy of the industry in its efforts to promote smoking, and to examine in detail the methods available to health workers and to governments for controlling the epidemic.

The issue should, we believe, serve as a resource for academics, a guide for health administrators, and as ammunition for the many active campaigners throughout the world who are seeking to bring an end to this tragic and preventable pandemic of disease and death.

We are most grateful to the experts, both from Britain and from several other countries, who have taken so much time and trouble to produce reviews on particular aspects. We also thank Dr Gill Haddock, the Managing Editor, who has so cheerfully and efficiently done so much of the editorial work; it has been a real pleasure to work with her.

John Crofton
Richard Doll
Scientific Editors

 ©The British Council 1996

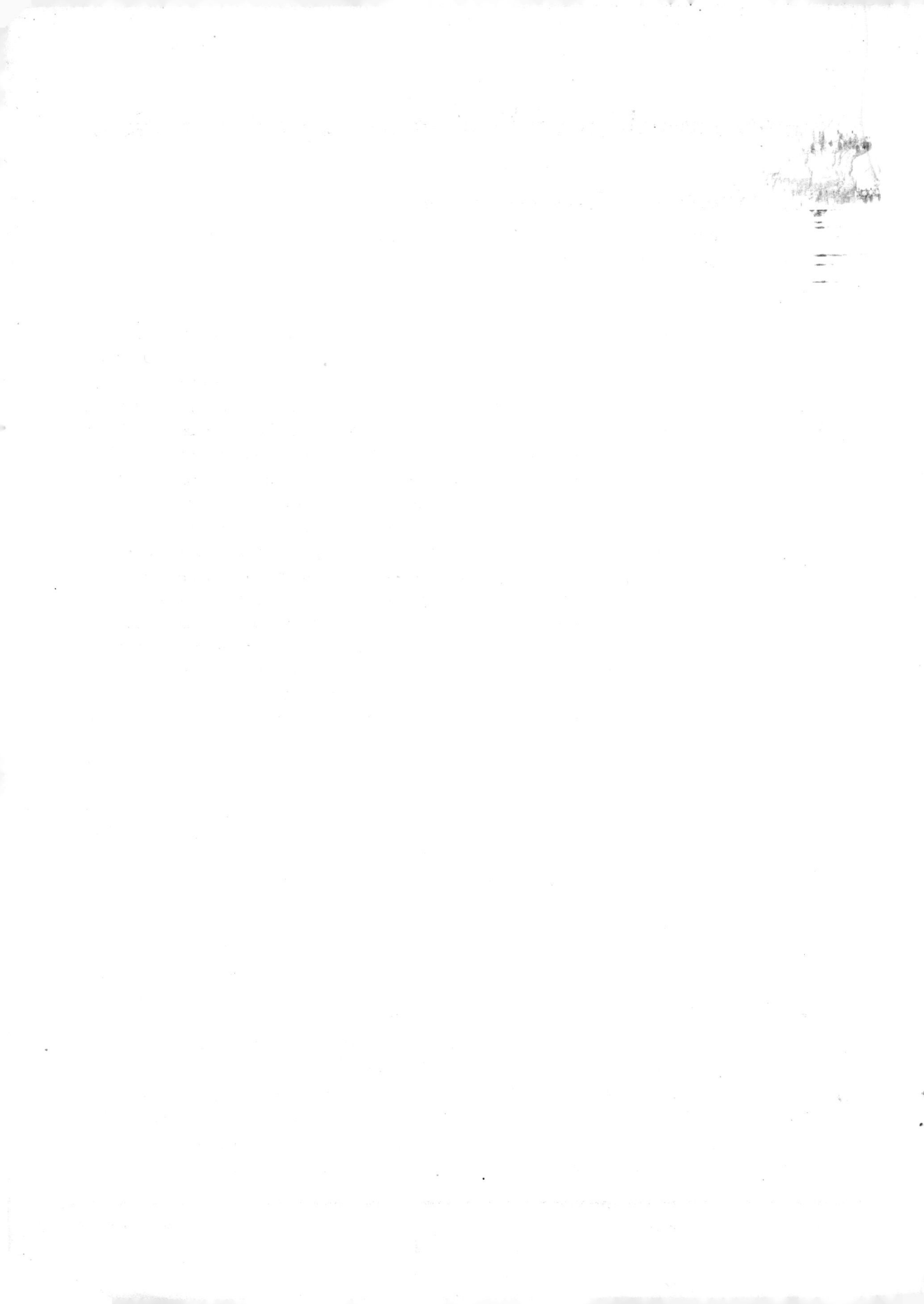

Cigarette smoking: an epidemiological overview

Nicholas J Wald* and **Allan K Hackshaw**

Department of Environmental and Preventive Medicine, Wolfson Institute of Preventive Medicine, The Medical College of St Bartholomew's Hospital, London, UK

The detailed mortality and morbidity statistics on smoking tend to conceal the overall impact of the habit on health. About 3 million people die each year from smoking in economically developed countries, half of them before the age of 70. Cancers of eight sites are recognized as being caused by smoking — lung cancer almost entirely and the others (upper respiratory, bladder, pancreas, oesophagus, stomach, kidney, leukaemia) to a substantial extent. Six other potentially fatal diseases are also judged to be caused by smoking: respiratory heart disease, chronic obstructive lung disease, stroke, pneumonia, aortic aneurysm and ischaemic heart disease, the most common cause of death in economically developed countries. Non-fatal diseases, such as peripheral vascular disease, cataracts, hip fracture, and periodontal disease, which cause appreciable disability, cost and inconvenience are also caused by smoking. In pregnancy, smoking increases the risk of limb reduction defects, spontaneous abortion, ectopic pregnancy, and low birth weight. While there are some diseases for which smoking shows a protective effect, the 'benefits' of these are negligible in relation to the illness and premature mortality caused by smoking. About 20% of all deaths in developed countries are caused by smoking; an enormous human cost which can be completely avoided.

Worldwide, about 3 million people currently die each year from smoking, half of them before the age of 70[1] — an enormous human cost. What is so unusual is the social and political acceptability of this lethal habit. The tobacco industry is probably responsible for more premature deaths and illness than any other organized commercial enterprise, exceeding the destructive impact of the arms and illicit drugs industries.

There are about 1 billion smokers in the world today, one-third of whom live in China. Table 1 shows the average number of manufactured cigarettes consumed per day per adult for 22 developed countries[2]. Smoking increased between 1945 and 1965 in all the countries, and from 1965 to 1985 it did not decline substantially in any of the countries and continued to increase in many. In 1985, 1650 billion cigarettes were sold in the countries listed in Table 1 — double the figure in 1955. Since 1985, there has been a decline in consumption in a few countries. In the UK, for example, the total number of cigarettes sold declined from 98 billion in

*Author for correspondence

©The British Council 1996

Table 1 Number of manufactured cigarettes consumed per day per adult (age 15 years or over) in 22 economically developed countries

	1945	1965 (relative to 1945)	1985 (relative to 1965)
Australia	1.6	7.3 (4.5)	6.3 (0.9)
Austria	1.3	5.3 (4.1)	6.9 (1.3)
Belgium	1.1	5.4 (4.9)	5.4 (1.0)
Canada	4.5	9.0 (2.0)	8.1 (0.9)
Denmark	1.1	4.1 (3.7)	5.1 (1.2)
Finland	2.1	5.4 (2.6)	4.7 (0.9)
France	1.2	4.1 (3.4)	6.0 (1.5)
Germany	0.7[†]	5.8 (8.3)	6.4 (1.1)
Greece	2.3	5.3 (2.3)	9.7 (1.8)
Ireland	4.3	7.4 (1.7)	6.8 (0.9)
Israel	—	5.4[#] (—)	6.4 (1.2)
Italy	1.8	4.2 (2.3)	6.3 (1.5)
Japan	0.9	6.4 (7.1)	9.0 (1.4)
The Netherlands	1.3[‡]	5.6 (4.3)	3.8 (0.7)
New Zealand	2.7	6.3 (2.3)	6.3 (1.0)
Norway	0.6	1.4 (2.3)	1.9 (1.4)
Portugal	1.2	3.2 (2.7)	4.8 (1.5)
Spain	1.3	4.8 (3.7)	7.4 (1.5)
Sweden	1.3	3.7 (2.8)	4.5 (1.2)
Switzerland	3.2	8.5 (2.7)	8.1 (0.9)
UK	7.1	7.4 (1.0)	5.9 (0.8)
USA	7.0	10.5 (1.5)	8.7 (0.8)

[†] 1948
[‡] 1946
[#] 1967
Data taken from reference 2.

1985 to just over 93 billion in 1992/93[3]. Consumption figures for economically developing countries are not readily available, but the increase in consumption of cigarettes in many of these countries has been substantial over the past 30 years. For example, in China about 700 cigarettes per adult were consumed in 1970. This increased dramatically to about 2000 per year in 1990/92 (A Lopez, personal communication).

This brief epidemiological overview covers the health effects of active cigarette smoking on the smoker and in pregnancy. In February 1985, the International Agency for Research on Cancer, part of the World Health Organization, convened a workshop which reported on tobacco smoking[4]. Since that report, new evidence has reinforced conclusions about diseases that were judged at that time to be caused by smoking. New evidence has also identified additional diseases caused by smoking (see *Cancers weakly related to smoking* in this issue).

In this chapter, we first examine **fatal** diseases that are positively associated with smoking, classifying them according to the extent to which the difference in incidence (or mortality) between smokers and non-smokers is a causal effect of smoking (Tables 2 and 3). We use three

Table 2 Fatal diseases positively associated with smoking — study of male British doctors[5]

Disease	Standardised mortality per 100,000 men/year		Relative risk (b/a)	Absolute excess risk per 100,000 men/year (b–a)	Attributable proportion[†] (%)
	Life-long non-smoker (a)	Current cigarette smoker (b)			
(i) Increased risk largely or entirely caused by smoking					
Cancer of:					
Lung	14	209	15.0	195	81
Upper respiratory sites	1	24	24.0	23	87
Bladder	13	30	2.3	17	28
Pancreas	16	35	2.2	19	26
Ischaemic heart disease	572	892	1.6	320	15
Respiratory heart disease	0	10	—	10	100
Aortic aneurysm	15	62	4.1	47	48
Chronic obstructive lung disease	10	127	12.7	117	78
(ii) Increased risk partly caused by smoking					
Cancer of:					
Oesophagus	4	30	7.5	26	66
Stomach	26	43	1.7	17	17
Kidney	9	13	2.1	4	25
Leukaemia	4	7	1.8	3	19
Stroke	152	203	1.3	51	8
Pneumonia	71	138	1.9	67	21
(iii) Increased risk due to confounding					
Cirrhosis of liver	6	32	5.3	26	—
Cancer of liver	7	11	1.6	4	—
Suicide	23	37	1.6	14	—
Poisoning	7	19	2.7	12	—
All diseases excluding those in category (iii)	907	1823	2.0	916	23
All diseases excluding those in categories (ii) & (iii)	612	1324	2.2	712	26

Results taken from reference 5.

[†]The proportion of all deaths from the specified disease attributable to smoking, assuming 30% of the population are current smokers and that all the excess risk in smokers is due to smoking. In Group (ii) the actual proportions will be somewhat less than those specified.

categories: (i) increased risk largely or entirely due to smoking; (ii) increased risk partly due to smoking; and (iii) increased risk due to confounding. We then consider **non-fatal** diseases under the first of these three categories (Table 4), disorders in pregnancy (Table 5), and finally diseases negatively associated with smoking (Table 6).

The International Agency for Research on Cancer (IARC) Report assessed the evidence on confounding and assigned the smoking related diseases to one of these three categories. For some smoking related diseases, such as lung cancer and peripheral vascular disease, the excess incidence or mortality is almost entirely caused by smoking. For most diseases, part of the association is likely to be attributable to confounding, as smoking is correlated with a number of dietary and other factors that also cause disease. In Table 2, for example, alcohol is

Table 3 Fatal diseases positively associated with smoking — American Cancer Society (CPSII). Men and women aged 35 years or more

| | | Standardised mortality per 100,000/year[#] | | | Absolute excess | |
		Life-long non-smoker	Current cigarette smoker	Relative risk	risk per 100,000 per year	Attributable proportion[†] (%)
(i) Increased risk largely or entirely caused by smoking						
Cancer of:						
Lung	M	24	537	22.4	513	87
	F	18	213	11.9	195	77
Upper respiratory sites	M	1	27	24.5	26	89
	F	2	10	5.6	8	58
Bladder and other urinary organs	M	18	53	2.9	35	36
	F	8	21	2.6	13	32
Pancreas	M	18	38	2.1	20	25
	F	16	37	2.3	21	29
Ischaemic heart disease	M	500	970	1.9	470	22
	F	386	688	1.8	302	19
Aortic aneurysm[‡]	M	24	98	4.1	74	48
	F	11	52	4.6	41	52
Chronic obstructive pulmonary disease	M	39	378	9.7	339	72
	F	21	216	10.5	195	74
(ii) Increased risk partly caused by smoking						
Cancer of:						
Oesophagus	M	9	68	7.6	59	66
	F	4	41	10.3	37	74
Kidney	M	8	23	3.0	15	37
	F	6	8	1.4	2	11
Cerebrovascular lesions	M	147	328	2.2	181	27
	F	236	434	1.8	198	20
(iii) Increased risk due to confounding						
Cancer of cervix	F	8	18	2.1	10	—
All diseases excluding those in category (iii)	M	788	2520	3.2	1732	40
	F	708	1720	2.4	1012	30
All diseases excluding those in categories (ii) or (iii)	M	588	2010	3.4	1422	42
	F	438	1179	2.7	741	34

Relative risks taken from the American Cancer Study (CPSII)[7].

[#]Calculated using the published relative risk, the mortality in the population aged $\geqslant$ 35 years[8] and assuming that 30% of the population are current smokers.

[†]The proportion of all deaths from the specified disease attributable to smoking, assuming 30% of the population are current smokers and that all the excess risk in smokers is due to smoking. In Group (ii) the actual proportions will be somewhat less than those specified.

[‡]Taken from American Cancer Society (CPSII)[7].

also a cause of stroke and oesophageal cancer, and smokers, on average, drink more alcohol than non-smokers. Alcohol also predisposes to falls and hip fracture (Table 4), as does lack of exercise, and smokers may on average exercise less. For diseases in which confounding plays a role, the effect of smoking and a confounding factor, such as alcohol, often tends to act synergistically so that those who do not smoke avoid most of the excess risk.

Table 4   Non-fatal diseases positively associated with smoking

Disorder	Incidence per 100,000/year[†] Life-long non-smoker	Current smoker	Relative risk	Absolute excess risk per 100,000/ year	Attributable proportion[†] (%)	Reference
(i) Increased risk largely or entirely caused by smoking						
Peripheral vascular disease (age 45–74 years)	150	300	2.0	150	23	11
(ii) Increased risk partly caused by smoking						
Cataracts (men aged 40–84 years)	247	543	2.2	296	26	12
Crohn's disease	5	15	2.1	10	25	13
Gastric ulcer (aged 20–61 years, Norway)	60	201	3.4	141	42	14
Duodenal ulcer (aged 20–61 years, Norway)	61	250	4.1	189	48	14
Hip fracture (aged ⩾ 65 years)	453	587	1.3	134	8	15
Periodontitis (aged 19–40 years)[Prevalence]	22,500	67,000	3.0	44,500	38	16

[†]The proportion of all deaths attributable to smoking, assuming 30% of the population are current smokers and that all the excess risk in smokers is due to smoking. In Group (ii) the actual proportion will be somewhat less than those specified.

Fatal diseases

Table 2, based on data on male British doctors[5], shows the mortality in cigarette smokers and life-long non-smokers. The relative risk and the absolute excess risk in cigarette smokers is given for each disease, together with the attributable proportion — the proportion of all deaths for each specified disease that is due to smoking. Cancers of eight sites (considering upper respiratory cancers [lip, tongue, mouth, pharynx and larynx] as one site) are recognized as being caused by smoking. The increased risks of cancer of the bladder and cancer of the pancreas are now considered to be largely due to smoking[6]. Six other diseases are judged to be caused by smoking, including ischaemic heart disease, the most common cause of death in economically developed countries. Smoking is responsible for much of the disease specified in categories (i) and (ii), for example, over 75% of deaths from lung cancer and chronic obstructive lung disease. Smoking causes more deaths from ischaemic heart disease than any other disease; about 35% of all the excess deaths for the diseases specified in Table 2 (320/916) per 100,000. Overall, the death rate in cigarette smokers from all the specified diseases is double that in life-long non-smokers.

Table 3 is similar to Table 2 but based on the American Cancer Society study of over 1 million men and women aged 35 years and over[7]. The results are similar to those from the British Doctors' study, although the relative risk for stroke is larger (2.2 compared with 1.3), probably because the men in the Doctors' study were older and the relative risk of stroke decreases in older men. The table shows that, for most diseases,

Table 5 Disorders in pregnancy positively associated with smoking

Disorder	Incidence per 100,000/year[†] Life–long non–smoker	Current smoker	Relative risk	Absolute excess risk per 100,000/ year	Attributable proportion[†] (%)	Reference
Congenital limb reduction defects (births)	41	87	2.10	46	25	17
Spontaneous abortion	13,838	17,712	1.28	3874	8	18
Ectopic pregnancy[#]	441	971	2.20	530	26	19

[†]The proportion of all deaths attributable to smoking, assuming 30% of the population are current smokers and that all the excess risk in smokers is due to smoking. The actual proportion will be somewhat less than those specified if not all excess is due to smoking.
[#]It is uncertain how much of the association is causal; at least part of it is likely to be due to confounding.

the relative risk in women is similar to that in men. The relative risk for cervical cancer is 2.1 but the increase in risk may be largely due to confounding[9]; number of sexual partners is associated with the risk of cervical cancer and there is a strong relationship between the number of partners and current smoking[10] (see also the chapter *Cancers weakly related to smoking* by R Doll in this issue).

Non-fatal diseases

Table 4, based on various sources, is similar to Tables 2 and 3 but relates to diseases associated with smoking that are not usually fatal. Some diseases, such as peripheral vascular disease, are recognised to be caused by smoking, but others, such as cataracts, which cause appreciable disability, are less recognised. The relative risk of hip fracture in smokers compared with non-smokers is modest (1.3) but the frequency of the disorder means that smoking accounts for many cases. Periodontal disease is the major cause of teeth loss in adults, affecting nearly a quarter of non-smokers. The risk in smokers is substantial (relative risk of 3) and smoking accounts for about 40% of all periodontitis in communities in which about one-third of adults smoke. Some of this increase in risk may be due to confounding, for example, smokers brushing their teeth infrequently, but it is likely that a major part of the association is causal.

Disorders in pregnancy

Table 5 shows three disorders positively associated with smoking. A rare but serious hazard is congenital limb reduction defects in which part or all of a limb can fail to develop; the risk with maternal smoking is double

Table 6 Diseases negatively associated with smoking

Disease	Incidence (or deaths) per 100,000/year		Relative risk	Reference
	Non–smoker	Current (or ever) smoker		
Parkinson's (deaths)	8	4	0.50	21
Ulcerative colitis	16	13	0.70	13
Alzheimer's (aged over 65 years)	8286	5667	0.70	22
Endometrial cancer (women over 60 years)	230	110	0.50	23
Pre-eclampsia (births)	507	331	0.65	24
Down's syndrome (births)	147	90	0.60	25
Uterine fibroids (women aged 25–39)	3473	2430	0.70	26
Vomiting during pregnancy (hyperemesis gravidarum)	864	517	0.60	26

that in non-smokers. Spontaneous abortion occurs in about 15–20% of all pregnancies and although the proportion attributable to smoking is modest (28% increase) it accounts for almost 4000 cases per 100,000 women who smoke. The risk of having an ectopic pregnancy is double that in smokers—as many as a quarter of cases may be caused by smoking if all the excess is causal.

It has also been demonstrated that babies of smoking mothers weigh, on average, 150–250 g less at birth[18]. The association has been shown to be causal since randomised trials of smoking cessation in pregnancy have shown that birth weight can be increased[18]. Smoking is an important hazard in pregnancy.

Diseases less common in smokers

Table 6 summarises diseases that show a negative association with smoking. Much of the evidence is summarised in Wald and Baron[20] (see also the chapter *Protective effects of tobacco* by J Baron in this issue). There is a remarkable consistency in the data on smoking and Parkinsonism[21]—smokers have about half the risk of non-smokers. Most of the reduction is probably causal; there are no grounds for concluding that bias or confounding explains the association and there is a plausible pharmacological explanation for the association; nicotine stimulates dopamine release, which can ameliorate the disease. Smoking also reduces the risk of endometrial cancer—probably because of the anti-oestrogenic effect of smoking[23], smokers again having about half the risk of non-smokers. The position on Alzheimer's disease is uncertain. The summary relative risk from eight case-control studies (0.78) and one cohort study (0.70) are not very different from unity, so bias or confounding could be an explanation, and even chance cannot be totally excluded.

Smoking probably has a protective effect on ulcerative colitis[13], which contrasts with the increased risk of Crohn's disease (Table 4). The effect is consistent, though modest in size; the relative risk in case-control studies is about 0.5 and in two cohort studies it is about 0.7. The latter estimate is cited in Table 6. It is not widely recognised that the birth prevalence of Down's syndrome is lower in women who smoke than in non-smokers; relative risk 0.60, 95% CI 0.44–0.81 (based on a review of five studies[25] and supplemented by a further unpublished study provided as a personal communication by G Palomaki). The most likely explanation is that smoking increases the risk of miscarriage and this has a disproportionate effect in Down's syndrome pregnancies compared with unaffected pregnancies.

Taken as a whole, the 'benefits' arising from the protective biological effects of smoking are quantitatively much smaller and considerably less serious than illness and premature mortality caused by smoking.

Conclusion

The detailed mortality and morbidity statistics on smoking tend to conceal the overall impact of the habit on health. In Britain, for example, about one-third of adults smoke and half of these smokers will die of the habit, over one-third before the age of 65 years. In 1995, the total number of deaths attributed to smoking is estimated as 150,000 in the UK, over half a million in the USA, and in all developed countries about 2 million[27]. About 20% of all deaths in these countries are smoking-induced. The overall morbidity is more difficult to quantify but many millions of people will suffer illness and disability due to smoking. While the trend in cigarette consumption in some countries such as the UK is downward, this is not so in many countries. In every continent of the world, the public health impact of cigarette smoking is immense — a pandemic that is completely avoidable.

References

1 Peto R, Lopez AD, Boreham J, Thun M, Heath C. *Mortality from Smoking in Developed Countries: 1950–2000*. Oxford: Oxford University Press, 1994
2 Nicolaides-Bouman A, Wald NJ, Forey B, Lee P. eds. *International Smoking Statistics*. Oxford: Oxford University Press, 1993
3 *UK Customs and Excise Annual Report 1992/93*. London: HMSO, 1994

4   International Agency for Research on Cancer. *Tobacco Smoking*. (IARC Monographs on the evaluation of the carcinogenic risk of chemicals to humans, Lyons, IARC 1986 No 38)

5   Doll R, Peto R, Wheatley K, Gray R, Sutherland I. Mortality in relation to smoking: 40 years' observation on male British doctors. *BMJ* 1994; **309**: 901–11

6   International Agency for Research on Cancer. *Cancer, Causes, Occurrence and Control*. Tomatis L. ed. Lyon: IARC Scientific Publications No 100, 1990

7   Surgeon General Report. *Reducing the Health Consequences of Smoking: 25 Years of Progress*. US Department of Health and Human Services, 1989. Publication No CDC 89-8411

8   Office of Population Censuses and Surveys. *Mortality Statistics: Cause, 1992*. (Series DH2, no 19). London: HMSO, 1993

9   Phillips AN, Smith GD. Cigarette smoking as a potential cause of cervical cancer: has confounding been controlled for? *Int J Epidemiol* 1994; **23**: 42–9

10 Wellings K, Field J, Johnson AM, Wadsworth J. *Sexual behaviour in Britain. The national survey of sexual attitudes and lifestyles*. London: Penguin, 1994

11 Surgeon General Report. *Consequences of Smoking: Cardiovascular Disease*. US Department of Health and Human Services, 1983 Publication no PHS 84-50204

12 Christen WG, Manson JE, Seddon JM, *et al*. A prospective study of cigarette smoking and risk of cataract in men. *JAMA* 1992; **268**: 989–93

13 Logan RFA. Smoking and inflammatory bowel disease. In: Wald NJ, Baron J. eds. *Smoking and Hormone Related Disorders*. Oxford: Oxford University Press, 1990: 122–34

14 Johnsen R, Forde OH, Straume B, Burhol PG. Aetiology of peptic ulcer: a prospective population study in Norway. *J Epidemiol Community Health* 1994; **48**: 156–60

15 Law MR, Wald NJ, Meade TW. Strategies for the prevention of osteoporosis and hip fracture. *BMJ* 1991; **303**: 453–9

16 Haber J. Smoking is a major risk factor for periodontitis. *Curr Opin Periodontol* 1994; 12–18

17 Czeizel AE, Kodaj I, Lenz W. Smoking during pregnancy and congenital limb deficiency. *BMJ* 1994; **308**:1473–6

18 Department of Health and Social Security. Fourth report of the Independent Scientific Committee on Smoking and Health. London: HMSO, 1988

19 Campbell O. Ectopic pregnancy and smoking: confounding or causality. In: Poswillo D, Alberman E. eds. *Effects of Smoking on the Fetus, Neonate and Child*. Oxford, Oxford University Press, 1992: 23–44

20 Wald NJ, Baron J. eds. *Smoking and Hormone Related Disorders*. Oxford, Oxford University Press, 1990

21 Marmot M. Smoking and Parkinson's disease. In: Wald NJ, Baron J. eds. *Smoking and Hormone Related Disorders*. Oxford, Oxford University Press, 1990: 135–41

22 Hebert LE, Scherr PA, Beckett LA *et al*. Relation of smoking and alcohol consumption to incident Alzheimer's disease. *Am J Epidemiol* 1992; **135**: 347–55 [Incidence of Alzheimer's taken as 7.5% in people aged 65 years and over. Weatherall D. Ed. *Oxford Textbook of Medicine* 2nd edn 1987, pp 21–43]

23 Ross RK, Bernstein L, Paganini-Hill A, Henderson BE. Effects of cigarette smoking on 'hormone related' disease in a Southern California retirement community. In: Wald NJ, Baron J. eds. *Smoking and Hormone Related Disorders*. Oxford, Oxford University Press, 1990: 32–54

24 Hall MH, Harper PV. Smoking and pre-eclampsia. In: Poswillo D, Alberman E. eds. *Effects of Smoking on the Fetus, Neonate and Child*. Oxford, Oxford University Press, 1992: 81–8

25 Cuckle HS, Alberman E, Wald NJ, Royston P, Knight G. Maternal smoking habits and Down's syndrome. *Prenat Diagn* 1990; **10**: 561–7

26 Ross RK, Bernstein L, Vessey MP, Henderson BE. Hyperemesis gravidarum, uterine fibroids, and endometriosis: effects of cigarette smoking on risk. In: Wald NJ, Baron J, eds. *Smoking and Hormone Related Disorders*. Oxford, Oxford University Press, 1990: 64–71

27 Peto R, Lopez AD, Boreham J, Thun M, Heath C. Mortality from tobacco in developed countries:indirect estimation from national vital statistics. *Lancet* 1992; **329**:1268–78

Mortality from smoking worldwide[a]

Richard Peto*, Alan D Lopez[†], Jillian Boreham*, Michael Thun[§], Clarke Heath Jr[§] and Richard Doll*

*ICRF/MRC/BHF Clinical Trial Service Unit & Epidemiological Studies Unit, Harkness Building, Radcliffe Infirmary, Oxford, UK, [†]Tobacco or Health, World Health Organization, Geneva, Switzerland, [§]Epidemiology Unit, American Cancer Society, Atlanta, Georgia, USA

[a]Adapted from Peto *et al.* (1994)[1]

Estimates are made of the numbers and proportions of deaths attributable to smoking in 44 developed countries in 1990. In developed countries as a whole, tobacco was responsible for 24% of all male deaths and 7% of all female deaths, rising to over 40% in men in some former socialist economies and 17% in women in the USA. The average loss of life for all cigarette smokers was about 8 years and for those whose deaths were attributable to tobacco about 16 years. Trends in mortality attributable to tobacco differed between countries. In some the mortality in middle age (35–69 years) had decreased by half in men since 1965; in others it was continuing to increase. In women, the proportion was mostly increasing, almost universally in old age. Mortality not attributable to smoking decreased since 1955 in all OECD (Organization for European Collaboration and Development) countries, by up to 60% in men and more in women. No precise estimate can be made of the number of deaths attributable to smoking in undeveloped countries, but the prevalence of smoking suggests that it will be large. In the world as a whole, some 3 million deaths a year are estimated to be attributable to smoking, rising to 10 million a year in 30–40 years' time.

For the past few decades it has been widely known in developed countries that tobacco is dangerous; but it is still insufficiently widely known how large these dangers are. This is partly because of the failure to take account of the very long delay, perhaps lasting several decades, between starting to smoke and its full effect and partly because of the failure to recognize the very many different effects that smoking may have. Studies that would provide a direct estimate of the proportion of deaths in each country that is attributable to smoking might in principle be straightforward, but would in practice be extremely costly and time-consuming. It is possible, however, to provide estimates of the number of deaths attributable to smoking in developed countries by an indirect method, based on published vital statistics, and to estimate very roughly the number that is likely to occur worldwide in the early part of the next century, based on the current smoking patterns of young people.

We have, therefore, provided, for those interested in public health, estimates of the proportion of deaths attributable to smoking in each of the major populations that are classed by the United Nations as 'developed' (including the 15 newly independent countries that constituted the former USSR), and rounded estimates of the numbers of deaths that may be expected worldwide in the next few decades, if smoking habits are unaltered. We also give, for the developed countries, the trends in the estimated death rates attributable to smoking and those that may be deduced for deaths due to other causes in the absence of tobacco. The data are presented in greater detail elsewhere[1].

Mortality in developed countries

Deaths attributable to smoking

To estimate the number of deaths attributable to smoking in each country we have, first, compared the national lung cancer mortality rates with the rates that have been observed among US non-smokers and used the **absolute excess mortality** from lung cancer as an indication of the extent to which that population was being damaged by tobacco. This is justified, because in developed countries lung cancer is very closely related to smoking and so seldom caused by any other factor among non-smokers. Secondly, we used this lung cancer excess as a guide to the **fractions of the deaths** from other causes that could be attributed to tobacco, calibrating this relationship by epidemiological evidence from the massive cohort study of a million men and women carried out by the American Cancer Society in the 1980s[2]. Details of the method are described elsewhere[3].

The number of premature deaths estimated in this way to occur as a result of smoking is enormous. In males, it amounted in 1990 to 24% of all deaths in all developed countries combined and 35% in middle age (defined for this purpose as 35–69 years of age). In females, the proportion amounted to 'only' 7% (or 12% at ages 35–69), but these proportions are increasing. Indeed, in the few countries where women have smoked cigarettes regularly for several decades, the proportion of female deaths that is attributed to tobacco is now approaching the male figure. In the US, for example, the proportions of the male and female deaths in 1990 that were attributed to tobacco are, respectively, 26 and 17%. Elsewhere, the number of female deaths now attributed to smoking is still relatively small, for few of the middle-aged or older women are regular cigarette smokers. In many countries (such as France, The

Table 1 Number and percentage of deaths attributed to smoking in OECD developed countries in 1990

Country	Number of deaths in thousands (% in parentheses)						
	Males			Females			
	Aged (years)		All ages	Aged (years)		All ages	
	35–69	70+		35–69	70+		
Australia	6.7 (28)	7.3 (21)	14.0 (22)	1.9 (15)	3.1 (8)	5.0 (9)	
Austria	4.0 (28)	3.6 (16)	7.5 (20)	0.6 (7)	1.5 (4)	2.0 (5)	
Belgium	7.9 (41)	8.6 (28)	16.5 (31)	0.7 (6)	0.6 (1)	1.2 (2)	
Canada	13.5 (35)	14.1 (24)	27.6 (27)	5.0 (23)	7.0 (11)	12.1 (14)	
Denmark	3.3 (32)	4.3 (22)	7.6 (25)	1.8 (27)	2.6 (11)	4.4 (15)	
Finland	2.6 (25)	2.7 (21)	5.3 (21)	0.2 (5)	0.5 (3)	0.8 (3)	
France	32.6 (32)	24.5 (16)	57.1 (21)	1.0 (2)	1.2 (1)	2.2 (1)	
Germany	52.0 (32)	43.3 (18)	95.3 (22)	6.2 (7)	10.4 (3)	16.5 (3)	
Greece	5.2 (33)	5.2 (17)	10.4 (21)	0.4 (5)	0.9 (3)	1.3 (3)	
Ireland	1.7 (31)	2.5 (24)	4.2 (25)	0.7 (20)	1.6 (15)	2.3 (16)	
Italy	37.8 (37)	34.9 (21)	72.7 (26)	2.7 (5)	7.4 (4)	10.1 (4)	
Japan	26.8 (16)	41.5 (16)	68.3 (15)	3.6 (4)	15.4 (6)	19.0 (5)	
Luxembourg	0.2 (34)	0.3 (25)	0.5 (27)	<0.1 (9)	<0.1 (1)	0.1 (3)	
The Netherlands	8.6 (38)	13.0 (32)	21.6 (32)	1.4 (11)	1.3 (3)	2.7 (4)	
New Zealand	1.4 (28)	1.7 (22)	3.1 (22)	0.7 (21)	0.8 (9)	1.4 (11)	
Norway	1.4 (21)	1.9 (12)	3.4 (14)	0.4 (12)	0.6 (3)	1.0 (5)	
Portugal	4.0 (21)	2.8 (9)	6.8 (13)	0.0 (0)	0.0 (0)	0.0 (0)	
Spain	20.5 (33)	19.4 (19)	40.0 (23)	0.0 (0)	0.0 (0)	0.0 (0)	
Sweden	2.1 (16)	3.2 (9)	5.3 (11)	0.7 (10)	1.3 (3)	2.0 (4)	
Switzerland	3.1 (31)	3.7 (18)	6.8 (21)	0.3 (6)	0.9 (3)	1.2 (4)	
UK	37.2 (35)	52.1 (27)	89.4 (28)	16.4 (24)	32.1 (13)	48.5 (15)	
USA	150.0 (36)	136.2 (23)	286.3 (26)	72.7 (28)	102.1 (14)	174.9 (17)	
All	423.5 (32)	427.8 (20)	851.3 (23)	117.7 (16)	191.6 (7)	309.3 (9)	

Netherlands and Sweden), however, there have been large absolute increases in cigarette use by young women in the past few decades, foreshadowing large increases in female mortality from the habit early next century. Individual figures for the 22 developed countries participating in the Organization for Economic Collaboration and Development (OECD) are shown in Table 1 for two age groups and all ages in both sexes and similar data are shown for the 22 countries formerly with socialist economies (FSE) in Table 2. In both sets it is assumed that no death is caused by smoking under 35 years of age. In fact, a few are so caused, but the numbers are small and do not affect the overall percentages. The high proportions of premature deaths attributable to tobacco that are shown in the tables lead to the conclusion that the average loss of life for those killed by tobacco in developed countries in 1990 was about 16 years (17 years in the countries with former socialist economies and 14 years in the OECD countries). Since about half of all regular smokers in developed countries are eventually killed by the habit, teenagers or young adults who become regular cigarette

Table 2 Number and percentage of deaths attributed to smoking in former socialist economies in 1990

Country	Number of deaths in thousands (% in parentheses)					
	Males			Females		
	Aged (years)		All ages	Aged (years)		All ages
	35–69	70+		35–69	70+	
Armenia	2.2 (38)	0.5 (13)	2.8 (23)	0.2 (6)	<0.1 (1)	0.3 (3)
Azerbaijan	2.7 (24)	0.5 (8)	3.1 (14)	0.0 (0)	0.0 (0)	0.0 (0)
Belarus	11.0 (39)	3.1 (16)	14.1 (26)	0.3 (2)	0.1 (<1)	0.4 (1)
Bulgaria	8.2 (30)	2.2 (7)	10.4 (17)	0.5 (3)	0.4 (1)	0.9 (2)
Czech Rep	13.3 (42)	6.1 (19)	19.4 (29)	1.4 (9)	1.5 (3)	2.9 (5)
Estonia	1.9 (38)	0.5 (15)	2.4 (26)	0.2 (6)	0.1 (2)	0.3 (3)
Georgia	2.8 (24)	0.7 (9)	3.5 (15)	0.1 (2)	<0.1 (<1)	0.1 (1)
Hungary	16.0 (41)	6.5 (19)	22.5 (29)	3.1 (14)	3.1 (7)	6.0 (9)
Kazakhstan	15.2 (43)	3.7 (22)	18.9 (28)	2.3 (12)	1.9 (6)	4.2 (7)
Kyrgyzstan	2.0 (28)	0.7 (17)	2.7 (17)	0.2 (4)	0.3 (5)	0.5 (4)
Latvia	3.3 (38)	1.0 (15)	4.3 (25)	0.3 (6)	0.3 (2)	0.6 (3)
Lithuania	3.8 (38)	1.4 (17)	5.2 (25)	0.2 (3)	0.4 (3)	0.6 (3)
Moldova (Rep)	3.5 (31)	0.7 (10)	4.3 (20)	0.3 (3)	0.3 (3)	0.6 (3)
Poland	44.6 (42)	15.3 (18)	59.9 (29)	5.1 (10)	4.4 (4)	9.5 (5)
Romania	19.6 (32)	4.2 (8)	23.8 (18)	2.2 (6)	0.8 (1)	2.9 (3)
Russian Fedn	191.9 (42)	48.6 (20)	240.5 (30)	16.4 (7)	19.3 (3)	35.7 (4)
Slovakia	5.8 (38)	1.9 (15)	7.7 (26)	0.3 (4)	0.4 (2)	0.7 (3)
Tajikstan	0.7 (14)	0.2 (6)	1.0 (5)	0.0 (0)	0.0 (0)	0.0 (0)
Turkmenistan	1.1 (22)	0.2 (6)	1.3 (9)	0.0 (0)	0.0 (0)	0.0 (0)
Ukraine	64.4 (40)	19.5 (17)	83.9 (28)	5.9 (6)	8.5 (4)	14.5 (4)
Uzbekistan	4.7 (20)	0.9 (5)	5.6 (8)	0.7 (5)	0.5 (2)	1.3 (2)
Yugoslavia (former)	19.4 (36)	6.3 (13)	25.7 (23)	2.0 (6)	1.6 (2)	3.6 (4)
All	441.2 (39)	126.3 (17)	567.5 (26)	42.1 (7)	44.4 (3)	86.5 (4)

smokers must be reducing their life expectancy by the substantial amount of about 8 years. An 8 year loss of life expectancy for cigarette smokers is also indicated by the most recent evidence from the 40 year study of smoking and death among British doctors[4].

Trends in mortality attributed to smoking and to other causes

Two further sets of estimates are of special interest. The first shows the trends over the whole of the second half of this century in the absolute death rates attributed to smoking in two age groups in each sex. To obtain these trends, estimates of the proportions of deaths attributable to smoking have been derived by the same method from the cause-specific mortality rates published for the years 1955, 1965, 1975, 1985 and 1990. For the purpose of predicting what is likely to happen in the future, the trends at ages 35–69 years are of greater interest, as the trends at

Table 3   Trend in mortality attributed to smoking by sex and age: various populations

Population	Age (yrs)	Annual mortality attributable to smoking per 1000									
		Males					Females				
		1955	1965	1975	1985	1990	1955	1965	1975	1985	1990
Finland	35–69	6.53	7.50	6.11	4.65	3.35	0.15	0.00	0.05	0.31	0.24
Hungary	35–69	2.56	3.72	4.41	7.09	8.48	0.32	0.45	0.45	1.02	1.29
Ireland	35–69	2.73	4.20	4.80	4.58	3.59	0.66	0.77	1.46	1.44	1.30
Portugal	35–69	0.70	1.19	1.76	2.06	2.47	0.00	0.00	0.00	0.00	0.00
UK	35–69	6.51	7.32	6.22	4.78	3.79	0.55	0.96	1.35	1.60	1.53
US	35–69	3.27	4.75	4.91	4.36	4.13	0.06	0.39	1.08	1.66	1.78
OECD* countries	35–69	2.83	4.03	4.08	3.58	3.24	0.09	0.28	0.54	0.79	0.80
FSE* countries	35–69	3.61	4.47	5.49	7.07	7.31	0.26	0.32	0.42	0.54	0.55
Finland	70–79	12.60	19.42	20.02	19.15	15.55	0.00	0.00	0.23	1.15	1.29
Hungary	70–79	3.25	10.29	17.94	19.44	17.80	0.45	2.10	2.95	3.41	4.25
Ireland	70–79	2.03	7.56	15.67	19.85	18.13	0.00	1.63	3.99	7.61	7.38
Portugal	70–79	1.82	2.33	3.91	6.29	7.36	0.00	0.00	0.00	0.00	0.00
UK	70–79	13.13	21.60	26.40	22.78	18.90	0.93	1.91	3.63	5.85	6.35
US	70–79	3.98	8.90	13.51	14.61	14.48	0.00	0.20	1.58	4.52	6.06
OECD* countries	70–79	4.41	9.47	14.32	14.22	13.09	0.13	0.51	1.23	2.52	3.21
FSE* countries	70–79	6.05	8.87	12.37	15.36	15.35	0.33	0.46	1.05	1.64	2.02

*Organization for Economic Collaboration and Development and Former Socialist Economy countries

older ages will be more dependent on changes that took place in the distant past and, in some countries, are also less reliable, because the causes of death will have been less fully investigated. Trends in both age groups and both sexes for selected countries and groups of countries are shown in Table 3. Those for the other countries studied are generally similar or less marked. In some, the mortality in men attributed to smoking has decreased substantially, notably in the UK and Finland, in both of which it has decreased by about half at ages 35–69 years since 1965 and by about a quarter at ages 70–79 years since 1975. In others, notably in Hungary and Portugal, the mortality attributed to smoking has increased throughout, or, in the older age group, to at least 1985. In women, small decreases in the younger age group have been seen in a few countries, notably in Ireland where the rate has decreased by over 10% since 1975, but the rate at older ages in countries where any substantial proportion of women has been smoking for more than two decades is almost universally continuing to increase. In OECD countries as a group, the trends have been similar to those in the US, except that there has been slightly more indication of a decrease in older men and a less marked increase in women, while the trends in the former socialist economy countries as a group have been broadly similar to those in Hungary.

Owing to the increasing size of the world population and the increasing proportion of old people, the increase in the number of deaths attributable to smoking is proportionately greater than the increase in the death rate attributable to it. The estimated increase in

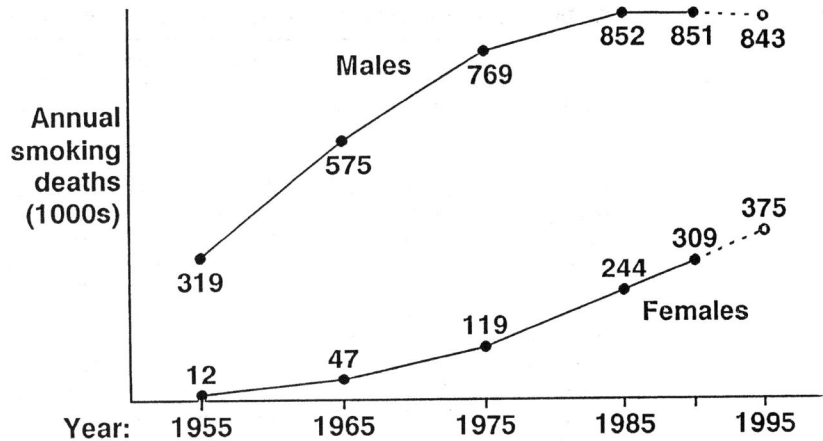

Fig. 1 Smoking-attributed numbers of deaths per year (all ages) in Organization for Economic Collaboration and Development countries[1,3]

deaths is shown in Figures 1 and 2, which give the numbers for 6 years between 1955 and 1995 for each sex in, respectively, OECD and FSE countries, the last numbers (for 1995) having been derived by extrapolation of the trends in the sex and age-specific death rates between 1985 and 1990.

The second set of estimates shows the trends in mortality that remain when the death rates attributed to smoking are subtracted from the overall death rates. These indicate what the underlying patterns might have been in the absence of tobacco. The results are given in Table 4 for the eight populations for which the trends in mortality attributable to smoking were shown in Table 3. In the OECD countries, the mortality in both age groups decreased by over 40% in men and by over 50% in women. Similar decreases occurred with minor variation in all the

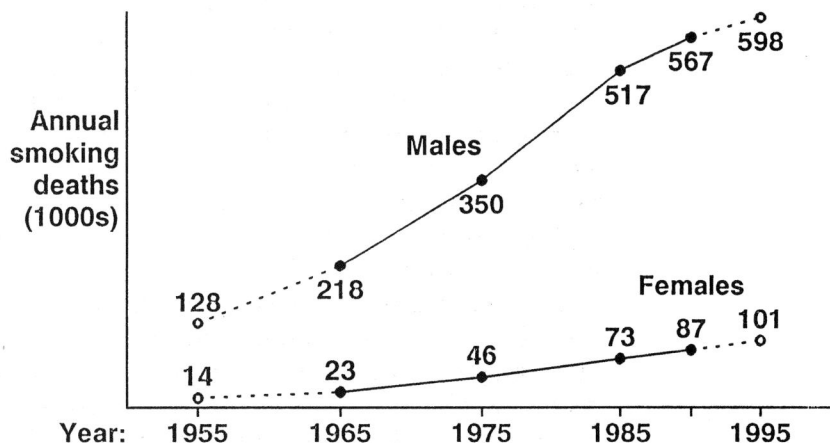

Fig. 2 Smoking-attributed numbers of deaths per year (all ages) in Former Socialist Economy countries[1,3]

Table 4 Trend in mortality not attributable to smoking by sex and age: various populations

Population	Age (yrs)	Annual mortality not attributable to smoking per 1000									
		Males					Females				
		1955	1965	1975	1985	1990	1955	1965	1975	1985	1990
Finland	35–69	13.24	11.99	11.21	9.50	9.30	9.84	8.82	6.65	4.99	4.75
Hungary	35–69	11.30	10.26	11.27	12.50	12.28	9.81	8.26	8.14	8.11	7.76
Ireland	35–69	11.75	10.07	9.51	8.38	7.90	10.12	8.06	6.88	5.59	5.01
Portugal	35–69	15.18	13.54	13.06	9.83	9.58	9.27	7.79	7.06	5.67	5.51
UK	35–69	9.34	8.23	7.98	7.34	6.93	8.33	7.01	6.13	5.22	4.73
US	35–69	12.92	11.97	9.57	7.62	7.06	9.16	8.25	6.10	4.84	4.40
OECD* countries	35–69	12.17	11.06	9.31	7.45	6.82	8.98	7.73	6.18	4.74	4.24
FSE* countries	35–69	14.05	10.64	11.67	11.92	11.48	10.00	7.56	7.74	7.94	7.50
Finland	70–79	82.48	73.79	61.73	55.50	50.85	71.79	69.45	48.65	38.68	35.31
Hungary	70–79	73.36	74.10	68.82	68.70	64.06	65.98	61.73	56.35	52.04	47.70
Ireland	70–79	80.54	68.83	62.49	60.45	52.77	70.77	56.73	48.49	38.53	33.19
Portugal	70–79	88.89	80.43	75.93	60.59	57.31	65.89	59.75	53.69	40.57	38.98
UK	70–79	75.22	62.44	56.00	49.86	45.66	57.45	48.78	41.99	34.67	30.58
US	70–79	67.48	63.35	53.59	44.85	40.29	50.74	44.72	35.95	28.94	25.55
OECD* countries	70–79	72.39	66.92	57.90	47.51	41.96	57.14	50.32	42.21	32.32	27.79
FSE* countries	70–79	69.47	60.42	61.69	68.13	62.35	53.43	48.15	48.42	51.28	46.73

*Organization for Economic Collaboration and Development and Former Socialist Economy countries

constituent countries, except that in Japan the mortality in men decreased by about 60% (61 and 57% in the two age groups) and by about two thirds in women (69 and 63% in the two age groups). In the former socialist economy countries, in contrast, the reduction was small (between 10–25%) and occurred principally in the first 10 years (1955 to 1965).

Modern medicine and the social conditions that a developed country can provide have not yet reduced mortality in middle age anywhere to the same extent that they have done in youth. The figures presented here, however, provide encouraging evidence that, in the absence of smoking, the achievements in many countries have been greater than is commonly thought. Death in old age is inevitable, but death before old age is not. In previous centuries, 70 years used to be regarded as humanity's allotted span of life and only about one in five survived to such an age. Nowadays, however, for non-smokers in 'OECD' developed countries, the situation is reversed. In the absence of tobacco, only about one in five will die before 70, and the non-smoker death rates are still decreasing, offering the promise of a world where death before 70 is uncommon.

Number of deaths attributable to smoking worldwide

In the present century, most of the deaths from smoking have been in developed populations, but next century the opposite will be true. The annual number of deaths from smoking is still increasing in the developed populations, but it will be increasing even faster elsewhere. There has, over the past few decades, been a massive global increase in cigarette consumption, which will have its chief effects on mortality in the next century. Estimates are therefore needed not only of the current health effects of past smoking patterns, but of the far larger future health effects of current smoking patterns. These were discussed in 1989 by a WHO collaborative group[5], the conclusions of which are summarised below.

Although more accurate information, particularly about the exact evolution of this epidemic, would still be very desirable, the order of magnitude of the current problem in developed countries has been reasonably reliably established. From Tables 1 and 2, the total number of deaths caused by tobacco was estimated to be over 1.8 million in 1990, so that, with allowance for an increased number of old people, tobacco must be expected to cause about 20 million deaths during the last decade of this century. At present most of these deaths from tobacco are male, but in many such countries female mortality from tobacco will eventually increase substantially as well, due to the large increases in female smoking over the past few decades.

For most developing countries the assessment of tobacco-attributable mortality is more difficult. Cigarette sales have increased substantially in recent years (much the largest absolute increase being in China), the male prevalence of smoking now exceeds 50% in many parts of the developing world (although the female prevalence is generally low), and chronic disease mortality rates are already high in many parts of Asia and Latin America. Overall, it was estimated that during the 1990s, the annual number of deaths from tobacco in the developing world would be about 1 million (including several hundreds of thousands in China, plus several hundreds of thousands in India and elsewhere), although this total is necessarily somewhat uncertain. When both developed and developing countries are taken together, tobacco is estimated to be responsible for an average of about 3 million deaths a year worldwide during the 1990s, with a range of uncertainty of perhaps 2–4 million.

At present there are 2.3 billion children and teenagers in the world and, on current smoking patterns, about 30–40% (i.e. about 0.8 billion) will be smokers in early adult life. A large recent prospective study in the US[2,3] indicated that, on average, persistent smokers have more than double the age-standardised death rates of lifelong non-smokers. If smoking caused a 2-fold excess at all ages it would eventually kill about half of all smokers. Not all the excess mortality associated with smoking is actually caused by smoking, however (although the greater part of it is), the mortality ratio beyond 75 years of age may be less than 2-fold, and the death rates from some unrelated causes (e.g. infectious diseases) are higher in developing countries than in the US. Consequently, the proportion of persistent smokers eventually killed by the habit in developing countries will probably be somewhat less than the proportion of about one-half that is suggested by the North American study. Even if the proportion is 'only' about one-third, however, then about 250 million of these 800 million future smokers will be killed by the habit.

If, on current smoking patterns, 200–300 million of those born in a 20-year period (e.g. 1970 to 1990) will be killed by tobacco, then at some stage around the middle of the next century (when the majority of these deaths will occur) the average annual number of deaths from tobacco must be about 1/20th of this, or about 10–15 million, and at some earlier stage the average annual number of deaths from tobacco will, therefore, be about 10 million. The uncertainty is not whether, but when, the annual total will, on present smoking patterns, be about 10 million – perhaps in the 2020s, but perhaps not until the 2030s. If the epidemic grows as rapidly in other developing countries as it seems to be doing in China[6], then the date might be earlier rather than later. Between 1978 and 1992, Chinese annual consumption of manufactured cigarettes increased from 500 billion to 1700 billion (about 30% of the world total) and cigarette tar levels were high; case-control studies in China have already shown large effects of prolonged smoking on the risk of lung cancer, and the 'background' death rates among non-smokers are already unusually high from diseases such as emphysema and cancer of the oesophagus (which suggests that among Chinese smokers the habit will cause particularly large hazards from these diseases). Indeed, the unpublished evidence from the nationwide 'spouse-control' study by Liu Boqi et al. of several hundred thousand Chinese deaths (plus the same number of controls) suggests that tobacco is already causing about half a million deaths a year in China, of which about half are due to chronic lung disease (Peto and Liu Boqi, personal communication).

If annual mortality from tobacco rises from about 3 million in the 1990s to about 10 million in the 2020s or early 2030s, then the average mortality over this 40-year period will be intermediate between 30–100 million per decade. Since most of those dying from smoking over the next 40 years (plus some of those dying from it more than 40 years hence) are already adults in 1990, about 200–300 million of today's 3 billion adults can be expected eventually to die from tobacco.

Combining the estimates for those now under 20 and for those now over 20 years of age, we estimate that, on present smoking patterns, about half a billion of the world's current population will eventually be killed by tobacco, and current experience in developed countries suggests that about half of them will be 35–69 years of age when killed. These predictions will be substantially wrong only if there are substantial changes in global smoking patterns.

References

1   Peto R, Lopez AD, Boreham J, Thun M, Heath C. *Mortality from smoking in developed countries*. Oxford: Oxford University Press, 1994

2   Garfinkel L. Selection, follow-up, and analysis in the American Cancer Society prospective studies. In: Garfinkel L, Ochs O, Mushinski M, eds. *Selection, follow-up, and analysis in prospective studies*. NCI Monograph 67. Bethesda: National Cancer Institute, 1985: pp 49–52

3   Peto R, Lopez AD, Boreham J, Thun M, Heath C. Mortality from tobacco in developed countries: indirect estimation from national vital statistics. *Lancet* 1992; 339: 1268–78

4   Doll R, Peto R, Wheatley K, Gray R, Sutherland I. Mortality in relation to smoking: 40 years' observations on male British doctors. *BMJ* 1994; 309: 901–11

5   Peto R, Lopez AD. The future worldwide health effects of current smoking patterns. 1990 report to the 7th World Conference on Tobacco or Health, on behalf of the WHO consultative group on statistical aspects of tobacco-related mortality. In: Durston B, Jamrozik K, eds. *The global war: Proceedings of the 7th World Conference on Tobacco or Health*. Perth: Health Department of Western Australia, 1990

6   Peto R. Tobacco: UK and China. *Lancet* 1986; ii 1038

Environmental tobacco smoke

Malcolm R Law and **Allan K Hackshaw**

Department of Environmental and Preventive Medicine, Wolfson Institute of Preventive Medicine, St Bartholomew's Hospital Medical College, London, UK

Environmental tobacco smoke is an important contaminant of indoor air. For a non-smoker living with a smoker the exposure is equivalent to about 1% of that from actively smoking 20 cigarettes a day (based on plasma cotinine). There is strong and consistent evidence that passive smoking increases the risk of lung cancer. It is estimated that there is an increase in risk of 24% (95% confidence interval 11–38%) compared to unexposed non-smokers, and several hundred lung cancer deaths per year in Britain are attributable to environmental tobacco smoke exposure. Passive smoking is associated with an increase in risk of chronic respiratory disease in adults of 25% (10–43%), and increases the risk of acute respiratory illness in children, by 50–100%. It is likely that passive smoking increases the risk of ischaemic heart disease, and that exposure in pregnancy lowers birthweight, but there is inconsistency between different estimates of the magnitude of risk. The overall hazard is sufficient to justify measures to restrict smoking in public places and workplaces, and to discourage people from smoking in their homes.

Environmental tobacco smoke is probably the most important contaminant of indoor air. It consists mainly of 'sidestream' smoke given off directly from the burning end of the cigarette; exhaled mainstream smoke is a minor component. The smoke differs in certain ways from active smoking: sidestream smoke is unfiltered (since it does not pass through the column of tobacco or the filter of the cigarette), and the nicotine is mainly in the gaseous phase in sidestream smoke and the particulate phase in mainstream smoke. These differences notwithstanding, it is reasonable to expect in general that environmental tobacco smoke exposure, or passive smoking, would cause the same diseases as active smoking, but at a risk reduced approximately in proportion to the considerable dilution of the smoke. This expectation is secure in the case of smoking-related cancers because of the evidence that carcinogens in general have no threshold. For other smoking related diseases there may plausibly be a threshold exposure level such that passive smoking constitutes too low a dose to convey any excess risk, or conceivably (though less plausibly) a near maximal response at low dose such that passive smoking conveys a risk of the same order of magnitude as active smoking.

©The British Council 1996

There is a reasonable basis for conducting epidemiological studies of exposure to environmental tobacco smoke for conditions in which the relative risk in active smokers compared to non-smokers is relatively large. In non-smokers married to smokers, the exposure to tobacco smoke is about 1% that of actively smoking 20 cigarettes per day[2,3] (based on concentrations of cotinine, the principal metabolite of nicotine). In the case of a disease for which actively smoking 20 cigarettes per day conveyed a 20-fold excess risk, the expected excess risk from passive smoking would be 20% (1% of 20) and the relative risk 1.2. This could be detected in a large epidemiological study (or a meta-analysis of several smaller studies). The difficulty in assessing and quantifying the health effects of environmental tobacco smoke is that for many other smoking-related diseases the expected increase in risk is not large enough to be detected in epidemiological studies. For several diseases the risk in those who smoke 20 cigarettes per day is about double that in lifelong non-smokers[1]. It would be hopeless to attempt to demonstrate the expected excess risk associated with passive smoking of 1% (1% of the excess risk of 100% associated with active smoking).

Simple measures of household exposure, assessing spousal smoking in studies of non-smoking adults or parental smoking in studies of children, are commonly used to define an exposed group in epidemiological studies of passive smoking. It is difficult to quantify exposure in the workplace and other environments using questionnaires. Spousal smoking is also indicative of exposure outside the home as it categorises a non-smoker as likely to be tolerant of environmental smoke and hence less likely to avoid it. Animal studies are available for some smoking related conditions but they cannot quantify the risk of disease from typical exposure levels in humans.

Evidence on specific diseases

The evidence on the association between passive smoking and the major smoking related diseases is discussed below. Two issues not discussed are the simple irritant effects of environmental tobacco smoke (important because they affect many people) and the fire hazards associated with smoking.

Lung cancer

The observation that carcinogens have no threshold indicates that inhaled tobacco smoke must increase the risk of lung cancer. A reasonable

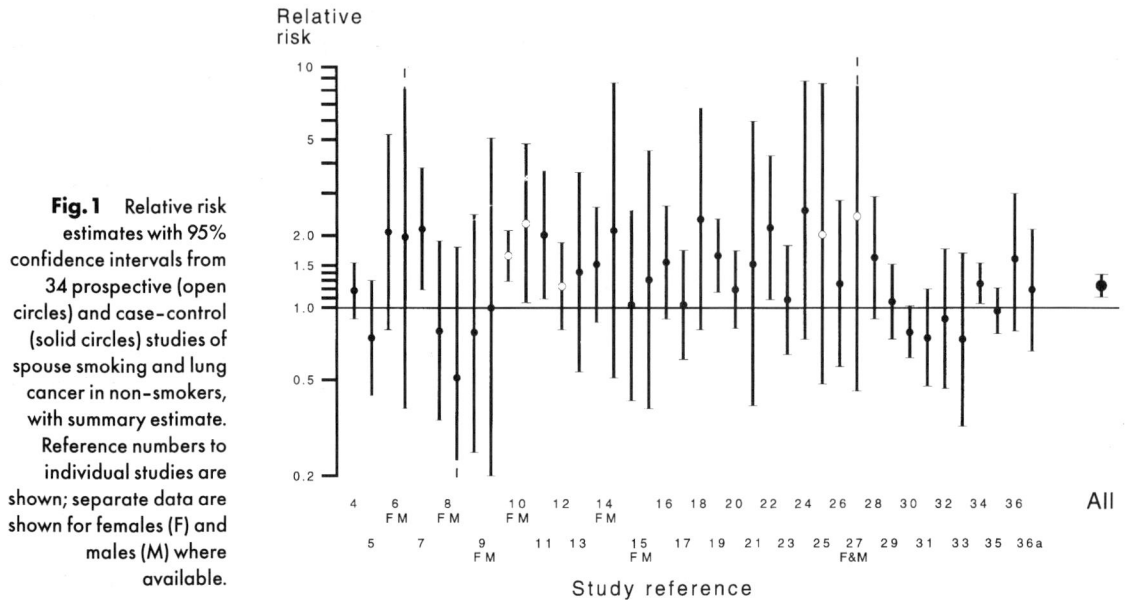

Fig. 1 Relative risk estimates with 95% confidence intervals from 34 prospective (open circles) and case-control (solid circles) studies of spouse smoking and lung cancer in non-smokers, with summary estimate. Reference numbers to individual studies are shown; separate data are shown for females (F) and males (M) where available.

expectation is that it will do so at a level proportional to the dilution. The last 20 years follow-up in the British Doctors Study demonstrated an excess risk of about 20-fold associated with actively smoking 20 cigarettes per day[1]. As discussed above, since the average exposure in passive smokers is about 1% that in active smokers of 20 cigarettes per day[2,3], the expected excess risk in non-smokers passively exposed, from linear dosimetry, would be 20%, and the relative risk 1.2.

Direct evidence from epidemiological studies confirms this estimate. Figure 1 shows the relative risk for spousal (or cohabitant) smoking in 34 published prospective and case-control studies of passive smoking and lung cancer[4–36a], updating an earlier published meta-analysis[37]. The combined relative risk estimate from all studies is 1.24 (95% CI 1.11–1.38; $p<0.001$). Figure 1 shows that the estimate from each individual study is consistent with the overall estimate, and that no one study is critical in influencing the combined estimate.

Biases in the epidemiological studies   There are two important biases in quantifying the risk. Misclassification bias arises because current smokers or former smokers, at increased risk of lung cancer, may falsely claim to be non-smokers. Smokers tend to marry other smokers, so these misclassified active smokers would be more prevalent in the group of exposed non-smokers than in the unexposed group, thereby spuriously increasing the risk estimate[37]. The second bias arises because individuals in the reference group, non-smokers living with non-smokers, are

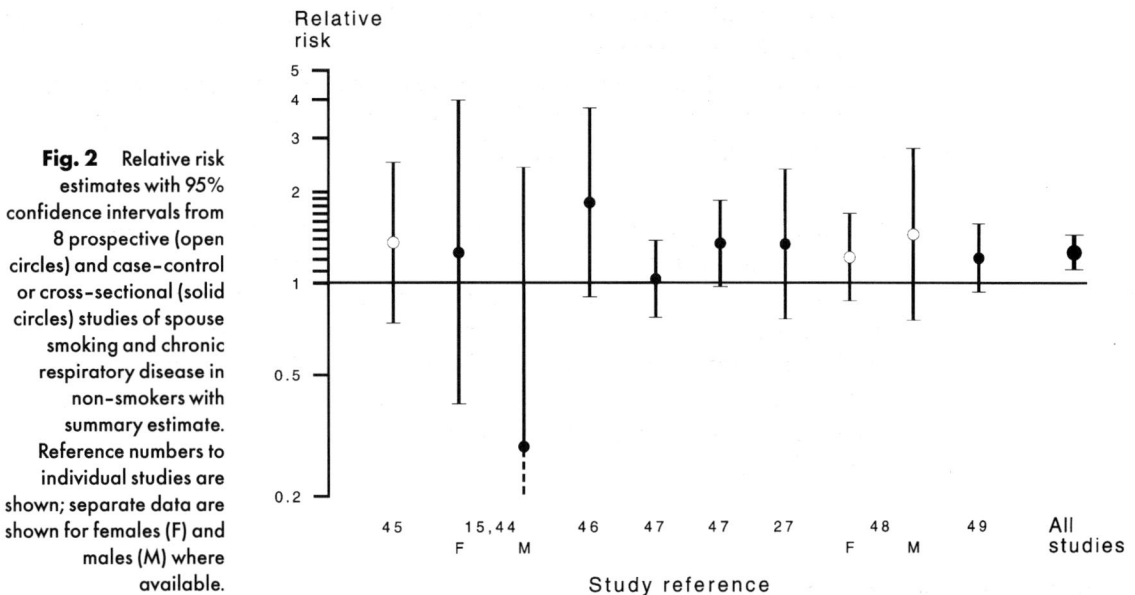

Fig. 2 Relative risk estimates with 95% confidence intervals from 8 prospective (open circles) and case–control or cross-sectional (solid circles) studies of spouse smoking and chronic respiratory disease in non-smokers with summary estimate. Reference numbers to individual studies are shown; separate data are shown for females (F) and males (M) where available.

estimate is consistent with a linear dosimetry estimate (1% of the excess risk of chronic respiratory disease in active smokers of 20 cigarettes per day). The conclusion that passive smoking causes chronic respiratory disease in adults is further supported by studies showing impaired lung function (peak expiratory flow rate and spirometry) in exposed compared to unexposed never-smokers[27,47,50,51].

Environmental tobacco smoke is irritant and likely to exacerbate asthma. However, there are few published data on adults shown to have asthma (reversible airways obstruction)[44,52], beyond the above studies in which the subjects mostly had chronic bronchitis and emphysema. There is by contrast a large body of evidence on asthma in children, discussed below.

Respiratory illnesses in children

Cotinine measurements have shown that infants and children whose parents smoke absorb the constituents of the environmental smoke[53,54]. As with adult non-smokers who live with smokers, the exposure is approximately equivalent to actively smoking one fifth of a cigarette per day[53]. Conclusions on environmental tobacco smoke and childhood illness are necessarily based on epidemiological studies alone, however; dosimetry calculations from studies of active smoking and adult diseases are inappropriate (see also the section by Charlton, page 98).

The epidemiological studies of parental smoking and childhood respiratory disease have been reviewed in detail by the US Environmental Protection Agency[52], whose documentation of the evidence is summarised here. The studies were considered in five groups. There is diagnostic overlap, and the first three groups might all be termed asthma.

Acute respiratory illnesses Review of 20 studies of acute respiratory illness in infants and older children (identified predominantly as hospital admissions with bronchiolitis or asthma) showed a greater risk in children exposed to tobacco smoke at home[52]. The association was independent of birthweight and socioeconomic factors. The evidence supports a cause-and-effect relationship. The risk associated with maternal smoking was greater than that with parental smoking, favouring a causal interpretation (since exposure to maternal smoking is greater[53], as infants spend more time with their mothers than their fathers) but inconsistent with an interpretation of confounding by social class (which should apply equally to both parents). Infants aged up to 6 months were at higher risk (about 3-fold) than older infants and preschool children (50–100% excess risk) while in older children the risk was smaller still; this declining effect with age also favours a causal interpretation, since infants spend more time at home with their mothers than older children.

Cough, sputum and wheezing Results of 26 studies of the prevalence of cough, sputum and wheezing in children showed that parental smoking increased risk, more so in infants (about two-fold risk) than school age children (about 50% excess risk)[52].

Asthma Ten studies have shown that passive smoking increases the frequency and severity of episodes of asthma in children who already have the disease, and increases the number of new cases (again by 50–100%)[52]. The demonstration of reduced lung function (spirometry and peak flow rate) in children of mothers who smoked, compared to children whose mothers did not smoke, supported the conclusion. The effect was not attributable merely to the irritant nature of tobacco smoke because decreased lung function was apparent long after the last exposure.

Acute and chronic middle ear disease Results of 15 epidemiological studies suggested that the association between parental smoking and middle ear disease was likely to be one of cause and effect[52,55], with an increase in risk of 50%. The finding of a linear dose-response relationship between salivary cotinine levels and the presence of abnormal tympano-metry was persuasive[55].

Sudden infant death syndrome   Eleven published studies have examined the effect of maternal smoking on the risk of sudden infant death syndrome (SIDS)[52,56], and together they show an approximate doubling in risk. In most of the studies, however, exposure was defined as maternal smoking during the pregnancy. While exposure is likely to continue after birth in almost all cases, it is difficult from such studies to distinguish the effects of exposure before or after birth. If one-third of women smoked during and after pregnancy, and smoking doubled the risk of SIDS, then 25% of all cases would be attributable to smoking; this 'attributable proportion' will decline as the prevalence of maternal smoking during and after pregnancy declines.

Conclusions   There is diagnostic overlap between the above five groupings, but the fact that a positive association was observed within each grouping weights against any diagnostic bias. The evidence strongly supports a conclusion that parental smoking increases the risk of respiratory illness in infancy and childhood. The consistent association in epidemiological studies (prevalence of illness increased by 50–100% in infants and preschool children) is confirmed by the stronger relationship with maternal than paternal smoking and in younger than older children, the linear relationship between cotinine and tympanometry and the demonstration of reduced lung function in children of parents who smoke.

Passive smoking in pregnancy

Active smoking by pregnant women reduces birthweight (by about 200 g on average) with an associated increase in perinatal mortality of about 28%[57]. In three studies comparing the birthweight of babies born to non-smoking women exposed and unexposed to other people's tobacco smoke, the difference in birthweight was 24 g[57]. This difference is greater than would be expected from linear dosimetry (reducing the above estimate of 200 g by the ratio of tobacco smoke exposure associated with passive and active smoking). The three studies may therefore have failed to adequately control for confounding factors. Despite this uncertainty, however, some effect is likely and the Independent Scientific Committee on Smoking and Health recommended the avoidance as far as practicable of exposure to other people's smoke during pregnancy[57].

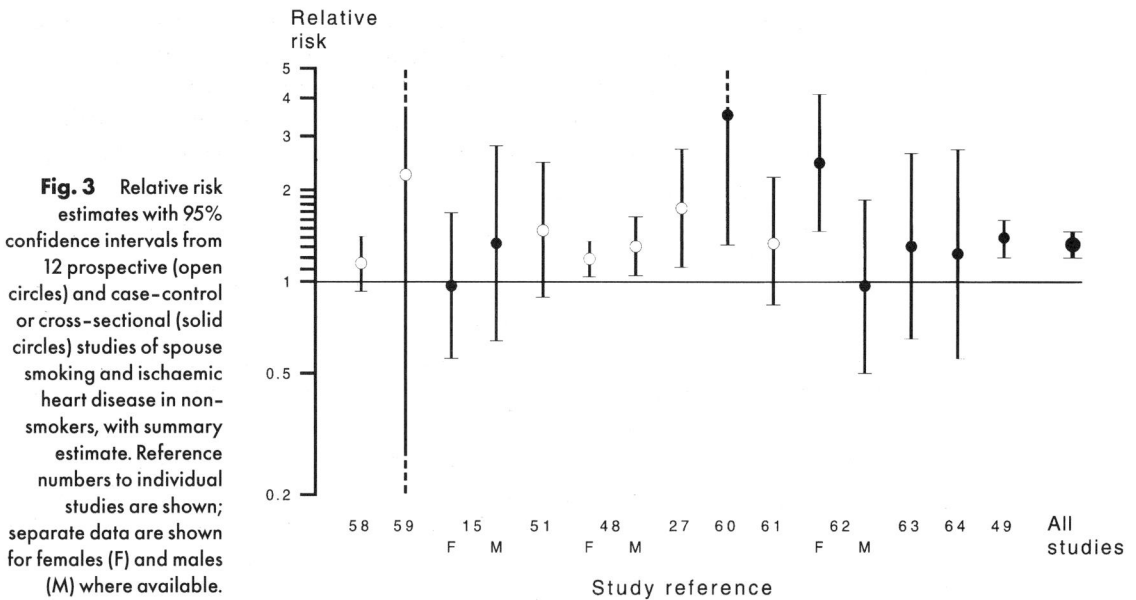

Fig. 3 Relative risk estimates with 95% confidence intervals from 12 prospective (open circles) and case-control or cross-sectional (solid circles) studies of spouse smoking and ischaemic heart disease in non-smokers, with summary estimate. Reference numbers to individual studies are shown; separate data are shown for females (F) and males (M) where available.

Ischaemic heart disease

The evidence on environmental tobacco smoke exposure and ischaemic heart disease (IHD) is difficult to interpret. Figure 3 shows the relative risk estimates from 12 prospective and case-control or cross-sectional studies of passive smoking and IHD[15,27,44,48,49,51,58–64]. The combined estimate is 1.3 (95% CI 1.2–1.4; $p<0.001$), and each individual study is consistent with this overall estimate of 1.3. The effect of the misclassification bias is negligible in the case of IHD because the relative risk with active smoking is much smaller for IHD than lung cancer.

Simple dosimetry considerations are inconsistent with this estimate of 1.3. Actively smoking 20 cigarettes per day approximately doubles the risk of IHD at the age of 60–65 years (the average age at death in the above 12 studies). It is implausible that an exposure equivalent to 1% of this should produce nearly half the mortality effect. The expected relative risk of IHD associated with passive smoking from linear dosimetry would be 1.01 (1% of the excess risk of 100%).

In view of this inconsistency, the association observed in the epidemiological studies might be attributed to confounding. Dietary antioxidant vitamins (markers for fruit and vegetable consumption) are associated with the risk of IHD in observational studies, the association is independent of serum cholesterol and other risk factors for IHD, and dietary intake of the vitamins differs between non-smokers married to smokers and to non-smokers[38,39]. Attributing all of the observed association to bias is as implausible as attributing it all to cause and effect, however, because it is difficult to envisage any confounding or other bias that would apply to passive smoking but not to active smoking. The dietary differences between smoking and non-smoking households would affect studies of active smoking as well as passive smoking. Attributing the relative risk estimate of 1.3 for passive smoking to dietary confounding implies that about half of the association with active smoking is also spurious. Yet a great deal of evidence indicates that this is not the case: the excess risk is largely reversed several years after stopping smoking for example. Also, experimental exposure of animals to environmental tobacco smoke has produced atheromatous disease[65,66], to an extent that would suggest a moderate increase in the risk of IHD in humans.

Glantz has proposed a causal mechanism whereby active and passive smoking might increase the risk of IHD to a similar extent[65,66]. It is likely that active smoking increases the risk of IHD in part by increasing platelet adhesiveness, and he cites evidence suggesting similar effects of passive and active smoking on platelet adhesiveness – a maximal response at very low exposure. This proposal cannot be definitively accepted, if only because of the absence of any evidence that the measurements of platelet adhesiveness reflect platelet behaviour *in vivo*, or of any epidemiological evidence directly relating these measures of platelet adhesiveness to the incidence of IHD. But they lend some support to an acceptance of the results from the epidemiological studies.

The best interpretation may be that the association is partly due to confounding (hence a small part of the association between active smoking and IHD is also due to confounding), and partly indicates a causal relationship (hence at least one mechanism whereby smoking increases the risk of IHD is maximal at very low dose). However, no definitive conclusion is possible.

Other smoking related diseases

Active smoking increases the risk of several other important conditions including stroke, aortic aneurysm, peripheral vascular disease, peptic ulcer, hip and other age related fractures, cataracts and periodontal disease. The mortality and morbidity attributable to these conditions is so great that an excess risk attributable to passive smoking of even 1 or 2% (as predicted from linear dosimetry) would be important. However, the direct data from epidemiological studies are too limited to support any conclusion[44]. The dosimetry may be non-linear – there could be a threshold effect with no excess risk at low dose, or there could be a maximal response at very low dose as has been proposed for IHD[65]. No conclusion can be made in relation to these diseases.

Conclusions

There is strong and consistent evidence that passive smoking increases the risk of lung cancer and the risk of respiratory diseases in children and in adults. Several hundred lung cancer deaths per year in Britain[57], and about 3,000 in the USA[52], could be attributable to environmental tobacco smoke exposure, as well as a great deal of morbidity from asthma in children. There is inconsistency between direct estimates and projected estimates from studies of active smoking based on dosimetry in the evidence relating to pregnancy and to ischaemic heart disease, but some effect is likely. The overall hazard is sufficient to justify measures to prohibit or restrict smoking in public places and workplaces, and health education campaigns to discourage people from smoking in their homes.

References

1 Doll R, Peto R, Wheatley K, Gray R, Sutherland I. Mortality in relation to smoking: 40 years' observations on male British doctors. *BMJ* 1994; **309**: 901–11
2 Wald NJ, Boreham J, Bailey A, Ritchie C, Haddow JE, Knight G. Urinary cotinine as marker of breathing other people's tobacco smoke. *Lancet* 1984; i: 230–1
3 Wald N, Ritchie C. Validation of studies on lung cancer in non-smokers married to smokers. *Lancet* 1984; i: 1067
4 Garfinkel L. Time trends in lung cancer mortality among nonsmokers and a note on passive smoking. *J Natl Cancer Inst* 1981; **66**: 1061–6
5 Chan WC, Fung SC. Lung cancer in non-smokers in Hong Kong. In: Grundmann E. ed. *Cancer Campaign, Vol 6, Cancer Epidemiology*. New York: Gustav Fischer, 1982: pp 199–202
6 Correa P, Pickle LW, Fontham E, Lin Y, Haenszel W. Passive smoking and lung cancer. *Lancet* 1983; ii: 595–7
7 Trichopoulos D, Kalandidi A, Sparros L. Lung cancer and passive smoking: conclusion of the Greek study. *Lancet* 1983; ii: 677–8
8 Buffler PA, Pickle LW, Mason TJ, Contant C. The causes of lung cancer in Texas. In: Mizell M, Corres P. eds. *Lung Cancer Causes and Prevention*. New York: Verlag Chemie. 1984: pp 83–99
9 Kabat GC, Wynder EL. Lung cancer in nonsmokers. *Cancer* 1984; **53**: 1214–21
10 Hirayama T. Cancer mortality in nonsmoking women with smoking husbands based on a large-scale cohort study in Japan. *Prev Med* 1984; **13**: 680–90
11 Lam WK. A clinical and epidemiological study of carcinoma of the lung in Hong Kong. MD Thesis, University of Hong Kong, 1985. (Data later published in: Larn TH, Cheng KK. Passive smoking is a risk factor for lung cancer in never smoking women in Hong Kong. In: Aoki *et al.* eds. *Smoking and Health*. Amsterdam: Elsevier, 1988: pp 279–81)
12 Garfinkel L, Auerbach O, Joubert L. Involuntary smoking and lung cancer: a case-control study. *J Natl Cancer Inst* 1985; **75**: 463–9
13 Wu A, Henderson BE, Pike MC, Yu MC. Smoking and other risk factors for lung cancer in women. *J Natl Cancer Inst* 1985; **74**: 747–9
14 Akiba S, Kato H, Blot WJ. Passive smoking and lung cancer among Japanese women. *Cancer Res* 1986; **46**: 4804–7

15 Lee PN, Chamberlain J, Alderson MR. Relationship of passive smoking to risk of lung cancer and other smoking-associated diseases. *Br J Cancer* 1986; **54**: 97–105

16 Koo LC, Ho JHC, Saw D, Ho C. Measurements of passive smoking and estimates of lung cancer risk among non-smoking Chinese females. *Int J Cancer* 1987; **39**: 162–9

17 Pershagen G, Hrubec Z, Svensson C. Passive smoking and lung cancer in Swedish women. *Am J Epidemiol* 1987; **125**: 17–24

18 Humble CG, Samet JM, Pathak DR. Marriage to a smoker and lung cancer risk. *Am J Public Health* 1987; **77**: 5989–602

19 Lam TH, Kung ITM, Wong CM *et al.* Smoking, passive smoking and histological types in lung cancer in Hong Kong Chinese women. *Br J Cancer* 1987; **56**: 673–8

20 Gao Y, Blot WJ, Zheng W *et al.* Lung cancer among Chinese women. *Int J Cancer* 1987; **40**: 604–9

21 Brownson RC, Reif JS, Keefe TJ *et al.* Risk factors for adenocarcinoma of the lung. *Am J Epidemiol* 1987; **125**: 25–34

22 Geng G, Liang ZH, Zhang AY, Wu GL. On the relationship between smoking and female lung cancer. In: Aoki *et al.* eds. *Smoking and Health.* Amsterdam: Elsevier, 1988: pp 483–6

23 Shimizu H, Morishita M, Mizuno K *et al.* A case-control study of lung cancer in non-smoking women. *Tohoku J Exp Med* 1988; **154**: 389–97

24 Inoue R, Hirayama T. Passive smoking and lung cancer in women. In: Aoki *et al.* eds. *Smoking and Health.* Amsterdam: Elsevier, 1988: pp 283–5

25 Butler TL. The relationship of passive smoking to various health outcomes among Seventh-Day Adventists in California. Dissertation, University of California, Los Angeles, 1988

26 Svensson C, Pershagen G, Klominek J. Smoking and passive smoking in relation to lung cancer in women. *Acta Oncol* 1989; **28**: 623–9

27 Hole DJ, Gillis CR, Chopra C, Hawthorne VM. Passive smoking and cardiorespiratory health in a general population in the west of Scotland. *BMJ* 1989; **299**: 423–7

28 Kalandidi A, Katsouyanni K, Voropoulou N *et al.* Passive smoking and diet in the etiology of lung cancer among non-smokers. *Cancer Causes Control* 1990; **1**: 15–21

29 Sobue T. Association of indoor air pollution and lifestyle with lung cancer in Osaka, Japan. *Int J Epidemiol* 1990; **19**: S62–S66

30 Wu-Williams AH, Dai XD, Blot W *et al.* Lung cancer among women in north-east China. *Br J Cancer* 1990; **62**: 982–7

31 Janerich DT, Thompson WD, Varela LR *et al.* Lung cancer and exposure to tobacco smoke in the household. *N Engl J Med* 1990; **323**: 632–6

32 Kabat GC. Epidemiologic studies of the relationship between passive smoking and lung cancer. *Washington, Winter Toxicology Forum* 1990: pp 187–99

33 Liu Z, He X, Chapman RS. Smoking and other risk factors for lung cancer in Xuanwei, China. *Int J Epidemiol* 1991; **20**: 26–31

34 Fontham ETH, Correa P, Reynolds P, *et al.* Environmental tobacco smoke and lung cancer in non-smoking women. A multicentre study. *JAMA* 1994; **271**: 1752–9

35 Brownson RC, Alavanja MCR, Hock ET, Loy TS. Passive smoking and lung cancer in nonsmoking women. *Am J Public Health* 1992; **82**: 1525–30

36 Stockwell HG, Goldman AL, Lyman GH *et al.* Environmental tobacco smoke and lung cancer risk in nonsmoking women. *J Natl Cancer Inst* 1992; **84**: 1417–22

36a Du YX, Cha Q, Chen YZ, Wu JM. Exposure to environmental tobacco smoke and female lung cancer in Guangzhou, China. *Proceedings of Indoor Air '93* 1993; vol. 1: pp 511–16

37 Wald NJ, Nanchahal K, Thompson SG, Cuckle HS. Does breathing other people's tobacco smoke cause lung cancer? *BMJ* 1986; **293**: 1217–22

38 Emmons KM, Thompson B, Feng Z, Hebert JR, Heimendinger J, Linnan L. Dietary intake and exposure to environmental tobacco smoke in a worksite population. *Eur J Clin Nutr* 1995, In press

39 Le Marchand L, Wilkens LR, Hankin JH, Haley NJ. Dietary patterns of female nonsmokers with and without exposure to environmental tobacco smoke. *Cancer Causes Control* 1991; **2**: 11–16

40 Dalager NA, Pickle LW, Mason TJ *et al.* The relation of passive smoking to lung cancer. *Cancer Res* 1986; **46**: 4808–11

41 Hecht SS, Carmella SG, Murphy SE, Akerkar S, Brunnemann KD, Hoffmann D. A tobacco-specific lung carcinogen in the urine of men exposed to cigarette smoke. *N Engl J Med* 1993; **329**: 1543–6

42 Trichopoulos D, Moll F, Tomatis L *et al.* Active and passive smoking and pathological indicators of lung cancer risk in an autopsy study. *JAMA* 1992; **268**: 1697–701

43 Darby SC, Pike MC. Lung cancer and passive smoking: predicted effects from a mathematical model for cigarette smoking and lung cancer. *Br J Cancer* 1988; **58**: 825–31

44 Lee PN. *Environmental Tobacco Smoke and Mortality*. Basel: Karger, 1992

45 Hirayama T. Non-smoking wives of heavy smokers have a higher risk of lung cancer: a study from Japan. *BMJ* 1981; **282**: 183–5

46 Kalandidi A, Trichopoulos D, Hatzakis A, Tzannes S, Saracci R. Passive smoking and chronic obstructive lung disease. *Lancet* 1987; **ii**: 1325–6

47 Kauffmann F, Dockery DW, Speizer FE, Ferris BG. Respiratory symptoms and lung function in relation to passive smoking: a comparative study of American and French women. *Int J Epidemiol* 1989; **18**: 334–44

48 Sandler DP, Comstock GW, Helsing KJ, Shore DL. Death from all causes in non-smokers who lived with smokers. *Am J Public Health* 1989; **79**: 163–7

49 Tunstall-Pedoe H, Brown CA, Woodward M, Tavendale R. Passive smoking by self report and serum cotinine and the prevalence of respiratory and coronary heart disease in the Scottish heart health study. *J Epidemiol Community Health* 1995; **49**: 139–43

50 Masi MA, Hanley JA, Ernst P, Becklake MR. Environmental exposure to tobacco smoke and lung function in young adults. *Am Rev Respir Dis* 1988; **138**: 296–9

51 Svendsen KH, Kuller LH, Martin MJ, Ockene JK. Effects of passive smoking in the multiple risk factor intervention trial. *Am J Epidemiol* 1987; **126**: 783–95

52 Office of Health and Environmental Assessment. *Respiratory Health Effects of Passive Smoking: Lung Cancer and Other Disorders*. United States Environmental Protection Agency, Washington DC, 1992

53 Jarvis MJ, Russell MAH, Feyerabend C *et al.* Passive exposure to tobacco smoke: saliva cotinine concentrations in a representative population sample of non-smoking schoolchildren. *BMJ* 1985; **291**: 927–9

54 Greenberg RA, Haley NJ, Etzel RA, Loda FA. Measuring the exposure of infants to tobacco smoke: nicotine and cotinine in urine and saliva. *N Engl J Med* 1984; **310**: 1075–8

55 Strachan DP, Jarvis MJ, Feyerabend C. Passive smoking, salivary cotinine concentrations, and middle ear effusion in 7 year old children. *BMJ* 1989; **298**: 1549–52

56 Nicholl J, O'Cathain A. Antenatal smoking, postnatal passive smoking and the Sudden Infant Death Syndrome. In: Poswillo D, Alberman E. eds. *Effects of Smoking on the Fetus, Neonate and Child*. Oxford: Oxford University Press, 1992: pp 138–49

57 *Fourth Report of the Independent Scientific Committee on Smoking and Health*. London: HMSO, 1988

58 Hirayama T. Passive smoking. *N Z Med J* 1990; **i**: 54

59 Garland C, Barrett-Connor E, Suarez L, Criqui MH, Wingard DL. Effects of passive smoking on ischemic heart disease mortality of nonsmokers. *Am J Epidemiol* 1985; **121**: 645–50

60 He Y, Li L, Wan Z, Li L, Zheng X, Jia G. Women's passive smoking and coronary heart disease. *Chin J Prev Med* 1989; **23**: 19–22

61 Humble C, Croft J, Gerber A, Casper M, Hames CG, Tyroler HA. Passive smoking and 20-year cardiovascular disease mortality among nonsmoking wives, Evans County, Georgia. *Am J Public Health* 1990; **80**: 599–601

62 Dobson AJ, Alexander HM, Heller RF, Lloyd DM. Passive smoking and the risk of heart attack or coronary death. *Med J Aust* 1991; **154**: 793–7

63 La Vecchia C, D'Avanzo B, Franzosi MG, Tognoni G. Passive smoking and the risk of acute myocardial infarction. *Lancet* 1993; **341**: 505–6

64 He Y, Lam TH, Li LS *et al.* Passive smoking at work as a risk factor for coronary heart disease in Chinese women who have never smoked. *BMJ* 1994; **308**: 380–4

65 Glantz SA, Parmley WW. Passive smoking and heart disease: epidemiology, physiology, and biochemistry. *Circulation* 1991; **83**: 1–12

66 Glantz SA, Parmley WW. Passive smoking and heart disease: mechanisms and risk. *JAMA* 1995; **273**: 1047–53

Cancers weakly related to smoking

Richard Doll

ICRF/MRC/BHF Clinical Trial Service Unit & Epidemiological Studies Unit, Radcliffe Infirmary, Oxford, UK

In 1985, review of the carcinogenic effects of tobacco led the International Agency for Research on Cancer to conclude that the smoking of cigarettes was an important cause of cancers of the lung, larynx, oro- and hypo-pharynx, oesophagus, bladder, renal pelvis, and pancreas and that the smoking of tobacco in other forms was also an important cause of some of them. More evidence about common cancers has now been obtained in cohort studies and about less common cancers in case-control studies. Many are weakly related to smoking. Review now justifies the conclusion that cigarette smoking is also a cause of cancers of the stomach, renal body, liver, and nose and of myeloid leukaemia and may be a cause of cancers of the nasopharynx and lip, and that pipe smoking is a cause of cancer of the lip. Associations between cigarette smoking and cancers of the large bowel and cervix uteri may be largely, and perhaps wholly, explained by confounding.

In February 1985, when a working group of the International Agency for Research on Cancer (IARC) met in Lyon to consider the carcinogenic effect of tobacco, it concluded that tobacco was carcinogenic to humans. In particular, it concluded that the smoking of cigarettes was an important cause of cancers of the lung, larynx, mouth, oropharynx, hypopharynx, oesophagus, bladder, renal pelvis, and pancreas, and that, for some of these cancers, the smoking of tobacco in other forms was also an important cause[1]. These conclusions were not difficult to reach, as the risk of developing each of these cancers had been found to be many times greater in heavy smokers than in lifelong non-smokers, the inhalation of tobacco smoke and the application of tobacco smoke condensate had been shown to cause cancer experimentally in animals, and similar conclusions had already been reached by some other expert committees (for example[2-6]). None of these conclusions has subsequently been seriously questioned and they are now generally accepted.

The evidence relating to several other types of cancer was also considered by the Agency. Cigarette smoking, it was concluded, was 'perhaps' an important cause of renal adenocarcinoma and it was noted that the risk of cervix cancer was increased in tobacco smokers and that associations had been found in some studies between smoking and cancers of the stomach and liver. The working group was, however, unable to conclude whether or not these last associations were causal in character.

In the 10 years that have passed since the Agency's review, much more evidence has been obtained about these last four types of cancer and also about several other types that were not specifically considered or mentioned in the group's conclusions and it is now evident that smoking is also a cause of several more cancers, if only a relatively unimportant cause. With weak associations, it is not to be expected that such direct evidence of causality can be obtained, as was obtained for lung cancer, when 95% of cases in men could be attributed to the habit. It should, nevertheless, not be thought surprising that smoking should be a cause of cancer in many different organs, for tobacco smoke contains a vast number of chemicals, some 50 of which have been shown to be carcinogenic in animals[1] and inhalation is a most effective way of getting a chemical into the systemic circulation and distributed throughout the body. Causation may, consequently, be deduced by analogy, if an association is consistently demonstrated between smoking and the development of a particular cancer and the observed association cannot readily be attributed to bias or confounding.

In this paper, I review the evidence relating to: (i) renal adenocarcinoma, which the IARC working group thought might 'perhaps' be caused by smoking; (ii) five common cancers that have been associated with smoking in large cohort studies: (iii) cervix cancer, which the IARC group noted was increased in incidence in smokers; and (iv) several rare cancers that can usefully be studied only by the case-control method.

Renal adenocarcinoma

Kidney cancer has consistently been found to be more common in cigarette smokers than in non-smokers, as, for example, in the large cohort studies of US veterans[7] and British doctors[8]. Cohort studies, however, have relied principally on death certificate diagnoses for classifying causes of death and have, in consequence, failed to provide separate evidence for the two principal types of the disease. For this we have to turn to case-control studies. These, at the time of IARC's 1986 review, provided such strong evidence of an association between smoking and transitional cell carcinomas of the renal pelvis that it was concluded that cigarette smoking was an important cause of that disease. The evidence relating specifically to adenocarcinoma of the renal body was, however, weak and, despite the fact that this histological type accounted for the great majority of all kidney cancers, the Agency concluded only that smoking was 'perhaps' a cause.

Since then, much more evidence has been obtained. All studies of more than 100 affected patients have found an increased risk in cigarette smokers compared to non-smokers. The risks have been small, seldom much more than 2-fold even in heavy smokers, and they have been much the same in many different countries: in Australia[9,10], Canada[11], China[12], Denmark[13], Italy[14,15] and the USA[16-20]. All, moreover, are compatible with the results of the collaborative study reported by McLaughlin *et al.*[21] which embraced 1774 patients and 2359 controls in Australia, Denmark, Germany, Sweden and the USA. These led to estimates of risk relative to that in lifelong non-smokers of 1.2 in ex-cigarette smokers, 1.1 in cigarette smokers smoking 1–10 a day, 1.3 in those smoking 11–20 a day, and 2.1 in those smoking 21 or more a day.

In this last study, and in several of the other smaller ones, adjustments were made for other factors for which there is substantial evidence that they might cause some cases of the disease (use of analgesics and thiazide diuretics and body mass index) without having any material effect on the estimated risk associated with smoking. N-nitrosodimethylamine, which has been shown to cause renal cancer in several animal species[22], has been found in tobacco smoke[1] and it can now be concluded that cigarette smoking is definitely a cause of adenocarcinoma of the renal body, as it is of transitional cell carcinoma of the renal pelvis.

Five common cancers associated with smoking

Five types of cancer have been consistently associated with smoking in cohort studies, other than those that the Agency concluded were caused by smoking (cancers of the stomach, colon, rectum, and liver, and leukaemia), renal adenocarcinoma, which has been considered above, and cervix cancer, which is considered below. The mortality from these cancers observed in four large cohorts is summarized in Tables 1 and 2, divided according to whether the subjects were lifelong non-smokers, ex-cigarette smokers, or continuing cigarette smokers smoking relatively small, moderate, or large amounts. For this purpose, cigarette smokers who were known also to have smoked pipes or cigars have been excluded.

In the smallest study, some 34,000 male British doctors were followed for 40 years[8]. The men's smoking habits had been determined in 1951 and again on four later occasions (in or shortly after 1957, 1966, 1971, and 1978) and deaths were related to the last known smoking habits. Altogether, 747 deaths were attributed to the five types of cancer in the five relevant smoking categories. In the second study, the smoking habits of some 400,000 American men and 600,000 American women were

Table 1 Relative risk of four cancers by smoking habit in 3 large cohort studies

Type of cancer	Study reference (sex)	No. of deaths†	Risk in cigarette smokers relative to lifelong non-smokers^a				
			Ex-	Current	Light	Moderate	Heavy
Stomach	8	168 (32)	1.0	1.7	1.6	1.7	1.7
	*(M)	353 (66)	1.6	2.1	2.0	2.1	2.4
	*(F)	217 (122)	1.4	1.4	1.5	1.0	1.5
	7	1058 —	1.0	1.4	1.3	1.4	1.7
	24	2839 (491)	—	1.5	1.4	1.5	1.5
Colon	8	246 (49)	1.4	1.3	1.3	1.1	1.4
	*(M)	1121 (279)	1.5	1.3	1.3	1.2	1.3
	*(F)	1082 (642)	1.0	1.1	1.3	1.2	0.7
	7	2596 —	1.4	1.2	1.1	1.2	1.5
	24	190 (45)	—	1.1	1.0	1.1	1.4
Rectum	8	85 (13)	1.4	2.3	1.3	1.9	4.4
	*(M)	172 (41)	1.2	1.5	1.1	1.7	1.5
	*(F)	156 (88)	1.0	1.6	1.5	2.1	1.1
	7	735 —	1.3	1.4	1.3	1.3	1.6
	24	254 (50)	—	1.4	1.3	1.4	1.4
Liver	8	51 (10)	1.4	1.6	2.4	0.4	2.2
	*(M)	198 (35)	1.7	2.5	1.8	2.6	3.0
	*(F)	101 (53)	2.1	1.6	1.0	2.0	2.1
	7	363 —	1.5	1.8	1.8	1.4	2.5
	24	652 (106)	—	1.5	1.6	1.4	1.7

^aRisks based on less than 10 deaths are underlined: †Number of deaths in non-smokers in parentheses. †Light, 1–14 a day, studies 8, 24 and *; 1–9 a day, study 7. Moderate, 15–24 a day, studies 8, 24 and *; 10–20 a day, study 7. Heavy, 25 or more a day, studies 8, 24 and *; unweighted mean 21–39 and 40 or more a day, study 7: *C Heath Jr (personal communication)

recorded by the American Cancer Society in 1982 and the subjects were followed for 6 years. Mortality rates are, however, given only for the last four to reduce the impact of including initially only self-reported healthy individuals. Altogether 2165 deaths in men and 1819 in women were attributed to the five cancers relevant to the five smoking categories. The findings, which were made available specifically for the purpose of this review (C Heath Jr, personal communication) pertain to cancer sites not examined in a detailed analysis published by the American Cancer Society[23]. In the third study, some 180,000 US veterans, who held government life insurance policies at the end of 1953 and were found to have been in one or other of the five selected smoking categories in 1954 or in response to further enquiry to non-responders in 1957, were followed to 30 September 1980[7]. Altogether, 5884 deaths were attributed to the five cancers listed in Tables 1 and 2. In the published report, mortality rates are given for four categories of continuing cigarette smokers, but they are reduced to three categories here by substituting the unweighted mean for the separate figures for men smoking 21–39 cigarettes a day and 40 or more cigarettes a day. Mortality is related to the men's smoking habits at the beginning of the study, which may have been up to 26 years before death occurred, so that the 'current smokers' for whom rates are given must be presumed to include a substantial proportion of men who had been ex-smokers for five or more years. In the fourth study, smoking habits were obtained from some 260,000 residents in six Japanese prefectures in 1966 and the subjects were followed for 16 years[24]. Altogether, 3935 deaths of men were attributed to the four cancers listed in Table 1. In the published report, mortality rates are given for five categories of regular cigarette smoker, but they are reduced to three by taking the means of the men smoking 1–4 and 5–14 cigarettes a day and smoking 25–34 and 35 cigarettes a day, weighted by the numbers of deaths in each group. The results for women are excluded, as very few Japanese women had smoked heavily for long. No data are given for ex-smokers.

Cancer of the stomach

In each of the four cohorts, the risk of stomach cancer in men is lowest in non-smokers, higher in current cigarette smokers, and highest in heavy cigarette smokers, while the risk in ex-cigarette smokers is equal to that in non-smokers or intermediate between the risks in non-smokers and current cigarette smokers in the three cohorts for which the data are given. In the one female cohort, the risk is greater in smokers than in non-smokers, but there are no similar gradients with continuity of smoking or amount. Similar findings to those in the four male cohorts have generally been obtained in the few other cohort studies and the many case-control studies that have now been reported from north and south America, Asia, Australasia, and Europe (see[1,25] for review and more recently[26,27]) although not infrequently, with relatively small numbers of cases, the excess in cigarette smokers has not been statistically significant (for example[28]). When all the data are examined, there can be no doubt about the reality of a positive association between cigarette smoking and the risk of the disease.

The association is, however, not necessarily causal and could be due to confounding, most obviously with a diet low in vegetables and fruit, and also with socio-economic status. Neither, however, seems to provide an adequate explanation for the results. For adjustment for dietetic factors has sometimes been possible and has not materially reduced the association, most notably in Hirayama's large cohort study in Japan[29], and similar relationships are seen in the socially homogeneous British doctors[8] and in the two large American studies of men employed in a wide variety of occupations[7,23].

No help can be obtained from ecological observations, as there have been major differences in the prevalence of the principal causes of the disease between different countries and at different times which would have overwhelmed the relatively small effect that, at the most, cigarette smoking could have caused. We have, therefore, to base our conclusion on the consistency of the findings, the dose-response relationship, the presence of chemicals in tobacco smoke that can cause gastric cancer in experimental animals, and the inability to explain the findings by confounding with other aetiological factors. On this basis, it is concluded that cigarette smoking is a minor cause of gastric cancer. As, however, tobacco smoke acts synergistically with whatever it is in food that causes gastric cancer, the absolute numbers attributable to smoking are large in areas where the risk of gastric cancer is high.

Cancers of the colon and rectum

Cancers of the colon and rectum are not always reliably distinguished on death certification or even in clinical records and, as they certainly have many causes in common and are often considered together in epidemiological studies as cancers of the large bowel, they are, for the most part, considered together here. There is, however, one important difference between them in the relationships shown in Table 1, for, whereas the mortality from rectal cancer is consistently greater in current cigarette smokers than in ex-smokers, this is not true for colon cancer.

Neither disease is consistently related to smoking in case-control studies[30] and a causal relationship has been postulated only on the basis of a *post hoc* hypothesis, based on the results of a cohort study[31] in which smoking was related to the presence of large polyps in the large bowel only when it had been continued for more than 20 years and with small polyps when it had been continued for less. Confounding is possible both with a high fat, low fibre diet[32,33] and with the consumption of alcohol[34], both of which have been related to the incidence of the disease [35,36] and confounding seems to be as likely an explanation of the associations observed in the cohort studies as causality.

Cancer of the liver

In developed countries, hepatocarcinoma, the principal type of liver cancer, nearly always occurs in association with alcoholic cirrhosis or with chronic infection with the hepatitis virus. The disease is consistently related to cigarette smoking, not only in the data shown in Table 1, but also in a large number of case-control and other cohort studies. Cigarette smoking, for its part, is closely related to the development of cirrhosis of the liver[8] and to the consumption of alcohol[34]. Quantitatively, the relationship between smoking and cirrhosis of the liver seems capable of being explained by the relationship between smoking and the consumption of alcohol and a simple explanation of the observed association between smoking and liver cancer is that it is due to confounding with the consumption of alcohol.

Cigarette smoking, nevertheless, is likely to contribute to the production of a few cases, for the smoke contains chemicals that are known causes of liver cancer in experimental animals (for example, methylnitrosourea) and both Hirayama[37] and Trichopoulos et al.[38] found that liver cancer was associated with cigarette smoking after adjusting for the consumption of alcohol. More importantly, smoking has been found to be associated with hepatomas in China in areas where little alcohol is drunk and infection with the hepatitis B virus is rare (L Boqi and R Peto, personal communication).

Leukaemia

Leukaemia had not been seriously considered as a disease that was contributed to by smoking until Austin and Cole[39] drew attention to the fact that the mortality from leukaemia had been increased in smokers compared to that in non-smokers in both the American Cancer Society's first cohort study of a million Americans[40] and Dorn's cohort study of some 250,000 US veterans[41]. Kinlen and Rogot[42] then examined the results of the veterans' study in greater detail and found that the mortality in cigarette smokers was significantly increased for leukaemia classed as

Table 2 Risk of leukaemia by smoking habit and cytological type in 3 large cohort studies

Type of cancer	Study reference (sex)	No. of deaths[†]	Risk in cigarette smokers relative to lifelong non-smokers[a]				
			Ex-	Current	Light	Moderate	Heavy
Myeloid	8	136 (7)	1.7	1.4	0.7	1.7	2.2
	*(M)	191 (47)	1.1	1.3	1.4	1.3	1.1
	*(F)	172 (103)	0.9	0.9	1.4	0.6	0.4
	41	281 (60)	1.5	1.7	1.3	1.8	1.9
Lymphatic	8	61 (17)	0.7	0.9	1.2	0.6	1.0
	*(M)	130 (35)	1.0	1.0	1.5	0.9	0.5
	*(F)	91 (51)	1.2	1.1	0.9	1.2	0.7
	41	181 (41)	1.6	1.6	1.4	1.8	1.5
All leukaemia	7	1132	1.3	1.3	1.1	1.4	1.3

[a]Risks based on less than 10 deaths are underlined: [†]Number of deaths in non-smokers in parentheses: [‡]Light, 1–14 a day, studies 8 and *; 1–9 a day, studies 7 and 41. Moderate, 15–24 a day, studies 8 and *; 10–20 a day, study 7 and 41. Heavy, 25 or more a day, studies 8 and *; 21 or more a day, study 41 and unweighted mean 21–39 and 40 or more a day, study 7. *C Heath Jr (personal communication)

lymphatic, myeloid or monocytic, or simply as acute, but that the increase was most marked for myeloid or monocytic and that it was only for this category that an increasing risk had been observed with increasing amount smoked. Table 2 shows Kinlen and Rogot's[42] results in comparison with those obtained specifically for myeloid and lymphatic leukaemia in the British doctors' study[8] and the later American Cancer Society's study (C Heath Jr, personal communication). Further data divided by cytological type have not been reported for the veterans' study, which Kinlen analysed, but the longer 26 year follow-up[7] has provided data for all leukaemia combined (now relating to over 1000 cases) and these latest follow-up results are also included in Table 2. The new data provide further evidence of a weak relationship between myeloid leukaemia and cigarette smoking in men but no evidence for a relationship in one study of women or between lymphatic leukaemia and smoking in either sex.

The results of a few other cohort studies and eight case-control studies have been reviewed by Bain[43] and these generally show similar relationships with smoking for myeloid and other non-lymphatic leukaemias and no relationship for lymphatic leukaemia in adults – either for the acute or the chronic type. That the relationship with myeloid leukaemia is real cannot be doubted. No other cause of leukaemia is known which could be confounded with smoking, while tobacco smoke contains two known leukaemogens: namely, radioactive isotopes of polonium and lead and benzene. The former, which derive principally from phosphate fertilisers, are minimal in amount (of the value of 0.01 Bq per cigarette, of which one fifth may be inhaled[1]) and the latter is likely to be the more important. According to Hoffman and Hoffman[44] the consumption of 20–40 cigarettes a day exposes a smoker to between 1–3 mg of benzene which, according to calculations made for the US National Institute for Occupational Safety and Health[45] might, over a 40-year period, increase the risk of leukaemia by about 10%. The calculation of risk per unit dose is, however, very uncertain, and other chemicals in smoke may prove to be equally or more important.

On the evidence now available, it can be concluded that myeloid but not lymphatic, leukaemia is another type of cancer that cigarette smoking may sometimes cause.

Cervix cancer

Cancer of the cervix uteri had been found to be associated with cigarette smoking so consistently in so many case-control and cohort studies that the IARC (1986) working group concluded that the association was certainly real[1]. They were unable, however, to decide whether the relationship was causal or due to confounding with a multiplicity of sexual partners. Quantitatively the increased risk in cigarette smokers was never large, commonly about 2-fold, and it was always reduced, though never eliminated, by adjusting for sexual activity with the rather crude indicators that used to be epidemiologically available. Now, however, that the risk of cervix cancer can be specifically related to infection with certain types of the human papilloma virus (HPV), it is possible to test for confounding directly by examining the relationship of cigarette smoking to the risk of infection. This has been done adequately only in one case-control study carried out in Spain and Colombia, the results of which show that the relationship with smoking does not hold in women positive for HPV types 16 and 18 (the two types most closely related to the development of this disease) but may continue to hold in women who are HPV negative[46]. The number of cases studied was, however, small and in each case the 95% confidence interval included unity.

Support for the idea that smoking might increase the risk of the disease is provided by the finding of mutagens in the cervical mucus of smokers but not of non-smokers[47] and by the reduction in the proportion of Langherhans' cells in the cervical mucosa of smokers[48]. Confounding, nevertheless, remains a plausible explanation of the findings, unless smoking can be shown to be significantly related to the disease after adjusting for infection with the carcinogenic types of HPV.

Rare cancers associated with smoking

Three types of cancer might be expected to be caused by smoking, as the organs in which they arise are exposed directly to tobacco smoke in the act of smoking: namely, cancers of the lip, nose, and nasopharynx. All are rare in developed countries and are more effectively studied by the case-control method than by following up cohorts.

Cancer of the lip

Lip cancer was the first type of cancer to be linked with smoking, when Sömmering[49] noted in a treatise for a prize offered by the Rhineland-Frankfurt Society, that 'carcinoma of the lip is most frequent when people indulged in tobacco pipes. For the lower lip is particularly attacked by carcinoma because it is compressed between the pipe and the teeth' (cited by Clemmesen[50]). In the first half of this century, as in the century before, lip cancer was relatively common; in recent years, however, it has become progressively less common, until by 1991–92 the mortality attributed to it in men was only about one tenth of that 40 years earlier, while that in women (now about 30% of that in men) had been reduced by about two-thirds. Some of the reduction is due to improved treatment, but much is due to reduced incidence. Now, less than 250 cases occur each year in the whole of England and Wales, about half the number that occurred in the early 1970s, when cancer registration was first established on a national basis.

No recent study has been reported, but seven studies were published between 1920 and 1970. Six showed a clear relationship with pipe smoking. Six provided estimates of relative risk for men who smoked only cigarettes, which were respectively nearly zero, 1.0, 1.4, 1.4, 2.4, and 2.6[6]. The two completely negative studies were published before 1945, whereas the others were published later, and the validity of the negative results may be questioned. There can be no doubt that the disease is caused by pipe smoking, nor that the effect is increased in outdoor workers with prolonged exposure to ultraviolet light[51]. There may also be some small contribution from cigarette smoking, but it remains to be proved.

Cancer of the nose

Cancers of the nasal cavity and nasal sinuses, commonly grouped together as cancers of the nose, occur only rarely throughout the world, apart from a few special situations in which people are heavily exposed at work to some specific carcinogenic substances. The most important of these have been situations in which men have been heavily exposed to some nickel compounds in the refining of nickel and to fine hardwood dusts in some sections of the furniture industry. Under these conditions the incidence of the disease has, on occasions, been increased several hundred-fold. Apart from these situations, which have, in total, caused only few cases and have had little impact anywhere on the national incidence of the disease, the incidence has been about twice as great in men as in women and has shown little or no change over the last few decades. The disease is, therefore, unlikely to be closely related to smoking.

In view of the known, and several other suspected, occupational hazards, the causes of the disease have been investigated in several case-control studies. Six have reported the relationship with cigarette smoking, five of which have found the risk in cigarette smokers to be increased. In the largest study, based on 175 patients with squamous carcinoma of the maxillary sinus in Japan, Fukuda et al.[52] found a significantly increasing trend with the amount smoked in 125 cases in men, with a relative risk of 4.6 in those smoking 40 or more cigarettes a day. For the 44 women, in whom no significant trend was found, detailed data were not given. In the two other studies based on more than 100 patients with cancer of the nose, only a small and non-significant increase of about 20% was observed for all cases in all cigarette smokers. Brinton et al.[53] however, found a significant increase (of 78%) for the 86 patients with squamous carcinomas and a significantly increasing trend with years of use and Zheng et al.[54] (who were unable to classify cases by histological type) found a significantly increasing trend with amount smoked per day and with duration of smoking and a significantly decreasing trend with years stopped.

Of the three smaller studies, one found relative risks of 1.6 for 92 patients with nasal cancers and 3.0 for the 50 patients with squamous carcinomas, with a significantly increasing trend with amount smoked and a significantly decreasing trend with time stopped in the latter group[55]. Another, with 60 patients, found a decreased relative risk for ever use of cigarettes of 0.7 but an increased risk of 1.6 in the 24 patients with squamous carcinomas[56], while the smallest study found a relative risk of 1.75 in 53 patients when those who had smoked 40 or more 'pack-years' were compared with those who had smoked 1 'pack-year' or less, which rose to 3.4 and was statistically significant in the 27 patients with squamous carcinomas[57].

For nasal cancer exceptionally, two studies have found a statistically significant association with exposure to environmental smoke. In a cohort study of 265,000 Japanese, Hirayama[58] found a relative risk of 2 in non-smoking women married to smoking men and, in a case-control study, Fukuda et al. found that the risk in non-smoking women increased with the number of smokers in the household[52]. The consistency of the results, the biological gradients observed with amount smoked and time since smoking stopped, and the experimental findings of nasal tumours in laboratory animals exposed to tobacco-specific nitrosamines[59] justify the conclusion that cigarette smoking is a cause of some squamous carcinomas of the nasal cavity and nasal sinuses, despite the small numbers studied. Also all methods of smoking are likely to contribute substantially to the risk of developing the disease through their contribution to environmental pollution. This, for physical reasons, could be relatively more important for the nose than for the lung.

Cancer of nasopharynx

Nasopharyngeal cancer is common in South China and some other areas in Asia and North Africa, where it has been shown to be dependent on infection with the Epstein–Barr virus and, in Chinese populations, with the consumption, particularly in childhood, of a special type of fish. Case-control studies in these areas and among Chinese migrants to the US have failed to show any consistent relationship with smoking, possibly because a small effect is masked by the much larger effects of viral infection and diet (see[60] for references).

In developed countries, the disease is everywhere rare, is about twice as common in men as in women, and has shown little or no change in incidence. It is, therefore, unlikely to be closely related to smoking. Only two substantial case-control studies have been carried out[61,62]. In one, which obtained an odds ratio of 1.0 for cigarette smokers, Chinese constituted 47% of the population of 156 affected patients and other Orientals 11%[61]. In the other, information about smoking habits was obtained for 204 white men and women who died from nasopharyngeal cancer in the USA and twice that number of controls, matched for sex and age, but otherwise drawn at random from a 1% sample of all who died in the country over the same period, excluding all whose deaths were thought to have been due to smoking-related diseases. The results gave odds ratios that increased with the amount smoked to levels of 3.1 for men and 4.9 for women with histories of 60 or more 'pack-years' of smoking. These findings closely resemble those obtained in the only other case-control study of a principally white population[63] and in the cohort study of US veterans[60]. The former, based on 39 cases and 39 matched controls, recorded an odds ratio of 2.8 for men and women whose maximum consumption had been greater than 1 pack a day. The latter, based on 48 cases, recorded odds ratios of 3.9 for current cigarette smokers, 1.5 for ex-cigarette smokers, and ratios that increased progressively from 1.8 for men smoking less than 10 a day to 6.4 (which was significantly greater than 1.0) for men smoking 40 or more a day.

The only other suspected cause in developed countries is occupational exposure to formaldehyde, which is present in tobacco smoke, and experimental studies have shown that tobacco specific nitrosamines can cause nasal cavity tumours in experimental animals[59]. Despite the small numbers on which the evidence is based, it can be concluded that cigarette smoking is probably a contributory cause of the disease.

Conclusion

Much more evidence about the effects of cigarette smoking has been obtained since 1986, when the International Agency for Research on Cancer concluded that it was an important cause of cancers of the mouth, oro- and hypo-pharynx, oesophagus, larynx, lung, pancreas, renal pelvis, and bladder[1]. It can now be concluded that cigarette smoking is also a cause of some cancers of the stomach, body of the kidney, liver, and nose, and of some myeloid leukaemias; probably a cause of some cancers of the nasopharynx; and possibly a cause of some cancers of the lip. It can also be concluded that pipe smoking has been a cause of many cancers of the lip in the past. Associations between cigarette smoking and increased risks of some other cancers (notably, cancers of the large bowel and cervix uteri) may be largely, and perhaps wholly, explained by confounding with other causative factors, but the possibility remains that cigarette smoking may also contribute to the causation of some cases in each site. The proportions of the additional cancers that are attributable to smoking are all small, but the absolute numbers that could be avoided by not smoking are substantial in areas where the background incidence of the disease is high, as is the case with gastric cancer in China and Japan. Although cigarette smoking is responsible for only small proportions of cases of renal adenocarcinoma and myeloid leukaemia it is still, on present evidence, the most important known avoidable cause of both.

References

1 International Agency for Research on Cancer. *IARC Monographs on the Evaluation of the Carcinogenic Risk of Chemicals to Humans: Tobacco smoking*. Vol. 38. Lyon: International Agency for Research on Cancer, 1986

2 Medical Research Council. Tobacco smoking and cancer of the lung. *BMJ*: 1957; **1**: 1523

3 Royal College of Physicians. *Smoking and Health*. London: Pitman, 1962

4 Royal College of Physicians. *Smoking and Health Now*. London: Pitman, 1971

5 Surgeon General. *Smoking and Health*. Report of the Advisory Committee to the Surgeon General of the Public Health Service. Washington: USDHEW, Public Health Services, US Government Printing Office, 1964

6 Surgeon General. *Smoking and Health*. Washington: USDHEW, Public Health Services, US Government Printing Office, 1979

7 McLaughlin JK, Hrubec Z, Blot WJ, Fraumeni JF. Smoking and cancer mortality among US veterans: a 26 year follow-up. *Int J Cancer* 1995; **60**: 190–3

8 Doll R, Peto R, Wheatley K, Gray R, Sutherland I. Mortality in relation to smoking: 40 years' observations on male British doctors. *BMJ* 1994; **309**: 901–1

9 McCredie M, Ford JM, Stewart JH. Risk factors for cancer of the renal parenchyma. *Int J Cancer* 1988; **42**: 13–16

10 McCredie M, Stewart JH. Risk factors for kidney cancer in New South Wales. I. Cigarette smoking. *Eur J Cancer* 1992; **28A**: 2050–4

11 Krieger N, Marrett LD, Dodds L, Hilditch S, Darlington GA. Risk factors for renal cell carcinoma: results of a population-based case-control study. *Cancer Causes Control* 1993; **4**: 101–10

12 McLaughlin JK, Gao Y-T, Gao R-N, Zheng W, Ji B-T, Blot W. Risk factors for renal cell cancer in Shanghai, China. *Int J Cancer* 1992; **52**: 562–5

13 Mellemgaard A, Engholm G, McLaughlin JK, Olsen JH. Risk factors for renal cell carcinoma in Denmark. I. Role of socio-economic status, tobacco use, beverages, and family history. *Cancer Causes Control* 1994; **5**: 105–13

14 Talamini R, Baron AE, Barra S *et al*. A case-control study of risk factors for renal cell carcinoma in northern Italy. *Cancer Causes Control* 1990; **1**: 125–31

15 La Vecchia C, Negri E, D'Avanzo B, Franceschi S. Smoking and renal cell carcinoma. *Cancer Res* 1990; **50**: 5231–3

16 Wynder EL, Mabuchi K, Whitmore WF. Epidemiology of adenocarcinoma of the kidney. *J Natl Cancer Inst* 1974; **53**: 1619–34

17 McLaughlin JK, Mandel JS, Blot WJ, Schuman LM. A population based case-control study of renal cell carcinoma. *J Natl Cancer Inst* 1984; **72**: 275–84

18 Asal NR, Risser DR, Kadamani S, Geyer JR, Lee EJ, Cheng N. Risk factors in renal cell carcinoma: 1. Methodology, demographics, tobacco use, and obesity. *Cancer Detect Prev* 1988; **11**: 359–77

19 Maclure M, Willett W. A case-control study of diet and risk of renal adenocarcinoma. *Epidemiology* 1990; **1**: 430–40

20 Hiatt RA, Tolan K, Queensberry CP. Renal cell carcinoma and thiazide use: a historical case control study. *Cancer Causes Control* 1994; **5**: 319–25

21 McLaughlin JK, Linblad P, Mellemgaard A *et al*. International renal-cell cancer study. 1. Tobacco use. *Int J Cancer* 1995; **60**: 194–8

22 Hamilton JM. Renal carcinogenesis. *Adv Cancer Res* 1975; **22**: 1–56

23 Thun MJ, Day-Lalley CA, Calle EE, Flanders WD, Heath CA. Excess mortality among cigarette smokers: changes in a 20-year interval. *Am J Publ Health* 1995; **85**: 1223–30

24 Akiba S, Hirayama T. Cigarette smoking and cancer mortality: risk in Japanese men and women – results from reanalyses of the six-prefecture cohort study data. *Environ Health Perspect* 1990; **87**: 19–26

25 Forman D. The etiology of gastric cancer. In: O'Neill IK, Chen J, Bartsch H, eds. *Relevance to Human Cancer of N-Nitroso Compounds, Tobacco Smoke and Mycotoxins*. IARC Scientific Publications No. 105. Lyon: International Agency for Research on Cancer, 1991

26 Hansson LE, Baron J, Nyren O, Bergstrom R, Wolk A, Adami HO. A population based case-control study in Sweden. *Int J Cancer* 1994; **57**: 26–31

27 Inoue M, Tajima K, Hitose K, Kutoishi T, Gao CM, Kitch T. Lifestyle and subsite of gastric cancer. *Int J Cancer* 1994; **56**: 494–9

28 Choi SY, Kahyo H. The effect of cigarette smoking and alcohol consumption in the etiology of cancers of the digestive tract. *Int J Cancer* 1991; **49**: 381–6

29 Hirayama T. Health effects of active and passive smoking. In: Aoki M, ed. *Smoking and Health*. Amsterdam: Elsevier, 1987

30 Baron JA, Sandler RS. Cigarette smoking and cancer of the large bowel. In: Wald N, Baron J, eds *Smoking and Hormone Related Disorders*. Oxford: Oxford University Press, 1990

31 Giovannucci E, Rimm EB, Stampfer MJ *et al*. A prospective study of cigarette smoking and risk of colorectal adenoma and colorectal cancer in US men. *J Natl Cancer Inst* 1994; **86**: 183–91

32 Thompson RI, Margetts BM, Wood DA, Jackson AA. Cigarette smoking and food and nutrient intakes in relation to coronary heart disease. *Nutr Res Rev* 1992; **5**: 131–52

33 Margetts BM, Jackson AA. Interactions between people's diet and their smoking habits: the dietary and nutritional survey of British adults. *BMJ* 1993; **307**: 1381–4

34 Doll R, Peto R, Hall E, Wheatley K, Gray R. Mortality in relation to consumption of alcohol: 13 years' observations on male British doctors. *BMJ* 1994; **309**: 911–18

35 Longnecker MP, Orza MJ, Adams ME, Vioque J, Chalmers C. A meta-analysis of alcoholic beverage consumption in relation to risk of colorectal cancer. *Cancer Causes Control* 1990; **1**: 59–68

36 Giovannucci E, Rimm EB, Stampfer MJ, Colditz GA, Ascherio A, Willett WC. Intake of fat, meat, and fiber in relation to risk of colon cancer in men. *Cancer Res* 1994; **54**: 2390–7

37 Hirayama T. A large scale cohort study on the relationship between diet and selected cancers of digestive organs. In: Bruce WR, Correa P, Lipkin M, Tannenbaum SR, Watkins TD, eds. *Gastrointestinal Cancer: Endogenous Factors* (Banbury Report 7). New York, Cold Spring Harbor, 1981

38 Trichopoulos D, MacMahon B, Sparros L, Merikas G. Smoking and hepatitis B-negative primary hepatocellular carcinoma. *J Natl Cancer Inst* 1980; **65**: 111–14

39 Austin H, Cole P. Cigarette smoking and leukaemia. *J Chron Dis* 1986; **39**: 417–21

40 Hammond EC. Smoking in relation to the death rates of one million men and women. In: Haenszel W, ed. *Epidemiological Approaches to the Study of Cancer and other Chronic Diseases*. National Cancer Institute Monograph 19. Bethesda: USDHEW, National Cancer Institute, 1966

41 Rogot E, Murray JC. Smoking and causes of death among US veterans: 16 years of observation. *Public Health Rep* 1980; **95**: 213–22

42 Kinlen LJ, Rogot E. Leukaemia and smoking habits among United States veterans. *BMJ* 1988; **297**: 657–9

43 Bain BJ. Does cigarette smoking cause leukaemia? *J Smoking Related Dis* 1986; **5**: 115–22

44 Hoffman D, Hoffman L. Recent developments in smoking-related research. *J Smoking Related Dis* 1995; **5**: 77–94

45 Rinsky RA, Smith AB, Horning R *et al*. Benzene and leukaemia. An epidemiologic risk assessment. *N Engl J Med* 1987; **316**: 1044–50

46 Muñoz N, Bosch FX, De SanJose S *et al*. Risk factors for cervical cancer in Colombia and Spain. *Int J Cancer* 1992; **52**: 750–8

47 Holly EA, Petrakis NL, Friend NF, Sarles DL, Lee RE, Flander LB. Mutagenic mucus in the cervix of smokers. *J Natl Cancer Inst* 1986; **76**: 983–6

48 Barton SE, Maddox PH, Jenkins D, Edwards R, Cuzick J, Singer A. Effect of cigarette smoking on cervical epithelial immunity: a mechanism for neoplastic change. *Lancet* 1988; **2**: 652–4

49 Sömmering ST. *De morbis vasorum absorbentium corporis humani*. Frankfurt: Varrentrapp and Wenner, 1795

50 Clemmesen J. *Statistical studies in malignant neoplasms. I. Review and results*. Copenhagen: Munksgaard, 1965

51 Doll R, Darby S, Whitley E. Trends in smoking related diseases. In: *The Health of Adult Britain*. London: Office of Population Censuses and Surveys, 1995: In press

52 Fukuda K, Shibata A. Exposure-response relationship between woodworking, smoking or passive smoking, and squamous cell neoplasms of the maxillary sinus. *Cancer Causes Control* 1990; **1**: 165–8

53 Brinton LA, Blot WJ, Becker JA *et al*. A case-control study of cancers of the nasal cavity and paranasal sinuses. *Am J Epidemiol* 1984; **119**: 896–906

54 Zheng W, Blot WJ, Diamond EL, Gao Y-T, Ji B-T. A population-based case-control study of cancers of the nasal cavity and paranasal sinuses in Shanghai. *Int J Cancer* 1992; **52**: 557–61

55 Hayes RB, Kardaun JWPE, de Bruyn. Tobacco use and sinonasal cancers: a case control study. *Br J Cancer* 1987; **56**: 843–6

56 Zheng, W, McLaughlin JK, Chow WH, Chien HT, Blot WJ. Risk factors for cancers of the nasal cavity and paranasal sinuses among white men in the United States. *Am J Epidemiol* 1993; **138**: 965–72

57 Strader CH, Vaughan TL, Stergachii A. Use of nasal preparations and the incidence of sinonasal cancer. *J Epidemiol Community Health* 1983; **42**: 243–8

58 Hirayama T. Cancer mortality in non-smoking women with smoking husbands based on a large-scale cohort study in Japan. *Prev Med* 1984; **13**: 680–90

59 Rivenson A, Furuya K, Hecht SS, Hoffman DD. Experimental nasal cavity tumors induced by tobacco-specific nitrosamines. In: Reznik HM, Stinson SF, eds. *Nasal Tumors in Animals and Man: Experimental Nasal Carcinogenesis*. Boca Raton: CRC Press, 1983

60 Chow WH, McLaughlin JK, Hrubec Z, Nam J-M, Blot WJ. Tobacco use and nasopharyngeal carcinoma in a cohort of US veterans. *Int J Cancer* 1993; **55**: 538–40

61 Henderson BE, Louie E, Jing JS, Buell P, Gardner MB. Risk factors associated with nasopharyngeal carcinoma. *N Engl J Med* 1976; **295**: 1101–6

62 Nam J-M, McLaughlin JK, Blot WJ. Cigarette smoking, alcohol and nasopharyngeal carcinoma: a case-control study among US whites. *J Natl Cancer Inst* 1992; **84**: 619–22

63 Mabuchi K, Bross DS, Kessler II. Cigarette smoking and nasopharyngeal cancer. *Cancer* 1985; **55**: 2874–6

Smokeless tobacco

Göran Pershagen

Institute of Environmental Medicine, Karolinska Institute, Department of Environmental Health and Infectious Diseases Control, Karolinska Hospital, Stockholm, Sweden

Smokeless tobacco practices are common in some parts of the world and the use seems to be increasing. Nicotine exposure is similar in smokeless tobacco users and smokers, often leading to strong physical dependence. As a rule, smokeless tobacco products contain high levels of nitrosamines with carcinogenic potency in experimental animals. Habitual use of oral tobacco can increase the risk of oral cancer, but the data are insufficient to assess in detail the risks associated with many types of smokeless tobacco. A recent study suggests that smokeless tobacco use is related to cardiovascular disease, which could be of great public health importance. The known and suspected health risks associated with the use of smokeless tobacco provide a basis for preventive action. In particular, efforts are needed to limit the introduction of such practices among young people, which may serve as a gateway to smoking.

Health risks related to smokeless tobacco have received comparatively little attention, in spite of widespread use in many parts of the world[1,2]. With the current emphasis on adverse health consequences of tobacco smoking, including exposure to environmental tobacco smoke, there may be a shift to increased use of smokeless tobacco. Such trends are already apparent in North America and Scandinavia[2,3]. Furthermore, smokeless tobacco practices may spread to populations and cultures where such habits are now rare. A few years ago, an attempt was made to introduce smokeless tobacco into the UK, with the intention of expanding to the European market. This resulted in a government ban and led, in due course, to a ban in the European Union except Sweden. Smokeless tobacco is also banned in Australia, Israel, Japan, Hong Kong, New Zealand, Saudi Arabia and Singapore[4].

This chapter focuses on health risks associated with smokeless tobacco. Initially an overview is given of the types of smokeless tobacco products used in different parts of the world, including time trends. Exposure to toxic agents in smokeless tobacco is taken up as a basis for the health risk assessment. The experimental and epidemiologic evidence on adverse effects of smokeless tobacco use is evaluated, with particular emphasis on cancer and cardiovascular effects. Most data relate to smokeless tobacco practices in Europe and North America. Thorough reviews of the health consequences of smokeless tobacco use have been performed by the

International Agency for Research on Cancer[1] and the US Surgeon General[2].

Uses

Smokeless tobacco is mainly used orally, and nasal use has become rare[1]. Chewing tobacco and snuff are the two major products in Europe and North America. Within these groups there are several types, differentiated by formulation and treatment of the tobacco. Chewing usually consists of placing a plug of tobacco in the gingival buccal area, where it is held or chewed. Many users chew tobacco during several hours a day.

Snuff is usually described as moist or dry[1]. Moist snuff is mainly used in Scandinavia and the US. In Sweden it is generally placed under the upper lip, while in Denmark the lower lip is preferred. In the US, the pinch is usually kept in the gingival buccal area. In some countries snuff is available in small packets wrapped in porous material, which appear to appeal to young adult users. Dry snuff is placed in the oral cavity or administered through the nasal passage.

The use of smokeless tobacco has increased in Scandinavia and the US in recent decades, particularly in teenagers and young adults[2,3,5]. In Sweden about 20% of boys aged 15 use snuff regularly, while the habit is much less common in girls[6]. 10% of Norwegian army conscripts aged 18–25 years reported daily use of moist snuff, and 23% were occasional users[7]. Smokeless tobacco practices are common in some parts of the US[2], in native Americans[8] and among athletes, such as baseball players[9]. The habits are particularly widespread among adolescent males, with national prevalence rates of about 5% for regular use and several times higher rates in certain regions[2].

Smokeless tobacco is also widely used in parts of Central and South-East Asia[1]. Tobacco may be used alone or in combination with other products, such as betel quid, ash and lime. In India, some forms are called khaini, mishri, zarda and kiwam, which constitute different preparations of tobacco (dried, roasted or boiled). The habit of nass is common in Central Asia with prevalence rates of up to 20% in some countries. Nass is usually made with local tobacco, ash and cotton or sesame oil, but the composition varies in different regions. Nasal snuff is widely used among the Bantu population in South Africa.

Exposure

More than 2000 chemical compounds have been identified in processed tobacco[1,2]. This includes original tobacco constituents and chemicals applied during cultivation, harvesting and processing. Major classes of compounds identified in tobacco include aliphatic and aromatic hydrocarbons, aldehydes, ketones, alcohols, phenols, amines, amides, alkaloids, metals and radioelements. Tobacco specific nitrosamines are formed from alkaloids during the processing of tobacco leaves. The concentrations in chewing tobacco and snuff may exceed by two orders of magnitude levels found in other consumer products. In recent years there seems to have been a decrease in the levels of tobacco specific nitrosamines in some products marketed in Sweden and the US.

The average consumption in regular users of snuff is about 10–15 g per day[1,10]. In general, the snuff is kept in the oral cavity during several hours per day. This holds true also for many other types of smokeless tobacco. Regular use often continues for decades.

Exposure to toxic agents in smokeless tobacco may be estimated from biological markers. Hemoglobin adducts of certain tobacco specific carcinogenic nitrosamines are substantially higher in snuff users than in smokers[11], indicating that systemic effects should be of concern. Measurements of nicotine and cotinine in blood indicate that nicotine exposure is comparable in smokeless tobacco users and smokers[2]. A recent Swedish study suggests that the nicotine intake may be higher in habitual snuff users than in smokers[12].

Cancer

Short term tests of genotoxicity provide information of some relevance for the cancer risk assessment. Various extracts of chewing tobacco can induce mutations, micronuclei, sister chromatid exchange and cell transformation[1]. Extracts of moist oral snuff can also produce mutations, sister chromatid exchange and chromosomal aberrations[13]. Khaini and nass are clastogenic[1], and a high mutagenic activity has been noted in the gastric fluid of chewers of tobacco with lime from India[14].

Carcinogenicity tests in experimental animals have been performed with different types of smokeless tobacco. Chewing tobaccos and extracts were tested by oral administration, topical application of the oral mucosa, subcutaneous administration and skin application in several rodent species[1,2]. In general, the investigations failed to demonstrate a significantly increased tumour production. The studies suffered from certain deficiencies, such as short application times and low dose exposures, which makes it difficult to evaluate the findings. Most tests with snuff also did not provide clear evidence of carcinogenicity[1,2], although effects were indicated in a recent study[15]. Results of combination treatments with other agents to assess tumour initiating and promoting activity are inconclusive. Some tobacco specific nitrosamines present in smokeless tobacco, such as N-nitrosonornicotine and 4-(methylnitrosamino)-1-(3-pyridyl)-1-butanone, are potent carcinogens in animal tests[1]. Oral administration produces carcinomas of the upper digestive tract and nasal cavity, while subcutaneous and intraperitoneal injection primarily induce tumours in the respiratory tract.

In the assessment of the epidemiologic evidence on carcinogenicity of smokeless tobacco, it is of interest to consider some local effects in the oral cavity. Oral leukoplakia is a common finding in snuff users, and is sometimes referred to as 'snuff dipper's lesion'[1,2]. It may in rare instances develop into a carcinoma, but is normally reversible following cessation of exposure. There is a close correlation between exposure (duration, intensity) and prevalence as well as severity of the lesions[16,17]. The prevalence of micronuclei and other nuclear anomalies is increased in the oral mucosa of snuff users[18,19], and the protein of the tumour suppressor gene p53 appears to accumulate in oral leukoplakias of snuff users[20].

A large number of case reports have described oral carcinomas in smokeless tobacco users, sometimes occurring at anatomic locations where the tobacco is routinely placed[1,2]. However, relatively few epidemiologic studies of high quality have investigated this relation. Most studies which do not specify in detail the type of smokeless tobacco used tend to show an association with oral cancer. For chewing tobacco 5 case-control studies provide no consistent evidence of an increased risk of oral cancer[1]. Methodological limitations in the studies make it difficult to interpret the findings.

A total of 6 case-control studies are available from Sweden and the US on oral snuff use and oral cancer[1,21] One early Swedish study indicated an increased risk of buccal and gum cancer in snuff users[22], while a recent study failed to show an effect for cancer of the head and neck region, including cancer of the oral cavity[21]. Three of the US studies provided evidence of an association between snuff usage and oral cancer[1]. In view of the high relative risks observed, confounding by smoking or alcohol use is unlikely as explanation for the findings. The most conclusive study showed a relative risk of 4.2 (95% confidence interval: 2.6–6.7) for oral and pharyngeal cancer in nonsmoking women from south-eastern US who used oral snuff, and a strong trend with duration of exposure for cancer of the gum and buccal mucosa[23,]. Cohort studies on snuff usage and oral cancer provide inconclusive evidence, but the interpretation is often difficult because of limited statistical power[1].

The data from Scandinavia and the US on smokeless tobacco and cancer of sites other than the oral cavity are relatively sparse[1,2,24,25]. Excess risks have been reported for carcinoma of the upper digestive tract and pancreas, but the evidence is not conclusive. A few studies on bladder cancer suggest that the risk is not altered to any large extent in users of smokeless tobacco products. Cohort studies from Scandinavia and the US indicate that the overall impact on cancer risk is much less in smokeless tobacco users than in smokers[1,26].

Several epidemiologic studies have been performed in relation to smokeless tobacco practices in Asia[1]. Use of tobacco plus lime (khaini) in India and Pakistan, as well as chewing betel quid containing tobacco, are associated with an increased risk of oral cancer. Relative risks exceeding 10 may be observed in regular users, indicating that a substantial proportion of the oral cancers are attributed to the exposure in populations where the habits are widespread. There is suggestive evidence for some other types of smokeless tobacco, such as nass. Specific mutations and overexpression of p53 protein are indicated in tobacco and/or betel chewing related oral carcinomas in India[27,28]. There is limited and inconclusive evidence on cancer risks following nasal snuff use in India and Africa[1].

Cardiovascular effects

Tobacco smoking is a major risk factor for cardiovascular disease and studies in smokeless tobacco users may help to elucidate the specific components responsible for this effect. Nicotine has pronounced acute effects on the cardiovascular system and gives rise to increased heart rate and blood pressure[2]. The time course of effects seems to be slower following oral snuff use than smoking.

The evidence is equivocal regarding effects by prolonged use of smokeless tobacco on cardiovascular risk factors. Increased blood pressure or hypertension rate in smokeless tobacco users was reported in some studies[29,30], while no effect was seen in others[31,32]. Similarly, results on hypercholesterolemia appear inconsistent[31-33]. A recent study indicates that snuff, unlike smoking, does not affect plasma fibrinogen levels[34].

Only two epidemiologic studies are available on smokeless tobacco and cardiovascular disease, and they both concern Swedish oral snuff users. A case-control study in northern Sweden showed an odds ratio for myocardial infarction of 0.89 (95% confidence interval 0.62–1.29) in nonsmokers, who used snuff daily[35]. On the other hand, smokers showed a clear increase in risk (odds ratio 1.87, 95% confidence interval 1.40–2.48). Blood pressure and serum cholesterol levels were similar in snuff users and smokers among the controls. A cohort study of Swedish construction workers revealed a relative risk for death from cardiovascular disease of 1.4 (95% confidence interval 1.2–1.6) in snuff users who had never smoked[26]. In smokers of ≥ 15 cigarettes/day who never used snuff the corresponding relative risk was 1.9 (1.7–2.2). The results were essentially the same when adjusted for cardiovascular risk factors, such as body mass index and blood pressure. A higher excess risk was indicated in those dying before 55 years of age in both snuff users and smokers. Tobacco habits were recorded at entry to the cohort, and subjects who took up smoking during the follow-up period may have contributed to the excess risk in snuff users. However, it is unlikely that this had a marked effect on the risk estimates.

Other health effects

Tobacco smoking is related to many types of health effects besides cancer and cardiovascular disease, which also could be of importance following smokeless tobacco use. Unfortunately, only few studies have investigated such effects. Most evidence relates to local lesions in the oral cavity. The role of smokeless tobacco for the development of gingivitis, parodontitis and dental caries remains equivocal[2]. There is a need for further studies on health risks associated with smokeless tobacco, particularly in populations where such habits are widespread. For example, a recent Swedish study suggests that use of oral moist snuff increases the risk of both Crohn's disease and ulcerative colitis[36], unlike smoking which increases the risk of Crohn's disease but ameliorates ulcerative colitis.

Conclusions

Smokeless tobacco practices are common in some parts of the world. The use seems to be increasing, for example in Scandinavia and the US. Nicotine in smokeless tobacco gives rise to strong physical dependence similar to tobacco smoking. Thus, habitual use of smokeless tobacco may serve as a gateway to smoking, which should be of particular concern among young people. In comparison to smoking, the evidence on health risks related to smokeless tobacco use is relatively limited. Habitual use of oral tobacco can increase the risk of oral cancer. The data are insufficient to assess in detail the risk associated with many types of smokeless tobacco products, but in some parts of the world the attributable proportion of oral carcinoma in regular users appears substantial. Effects on the cardiovascular system, such as myocardial infarction, are potentially of great public health importance. Unfortunately, available evidence is limited and inconclusive, and further studies are urgently needed. The overall health impact appears less from smokeless tobacco use than from smoking. However, the known and suspected health risks associated with smokeless tobacco indicate that it should not be viewed as an alternative to smoking.

References

1   *IARC Monographs on the Evaluation of the Carcinogenic Risk of Chemicals to Humans.* Vol 37, *Tobacco Habits other than smoking; betel quid and avoca nut chewing; and some related nitrosamines.* Lyon: International Agency for Research on Cancer, 1985

2   *The Health Consequences of Using Smokeless Tobacco.* A report of the advisory committee to the Surgeon General. Bethesda, MD: US Department of Health and Human Service, 1986

3   Nordgren P, Ramström L. Moist snuff in Sweden—tradition and evolution. *Br J Addict* 1990; **85**: 1107–12

4   Roemer R. *Legislative Action to Combat the World Tobacco Epidemic.* Geneva: World Health Organization, 1993

5   Giovino GA, Schooley MW, Zhu BP *et al.* Surveillance for selected tobacco-use behaviours– United States, 1990–1994. *Morb Mort Week Rep* 1994; **43**: 1–43

6   *Public Health Report 1994.* Stockholm: National Swedish Board of Health and Welfare

7   Schei E, Fönnebö V, Aaro LE. Use of smokeless tobacco among conscripts: A cross-sectional study of Norwegian army conscripts. *Prev Med* 1990; **19**: 667–74

8   Bruerd B. Smokeless tobacco use among Native American school children. *Public Health Rep* 1990; **105**: 196–201

9   Wisniewski JF, Bartolucci AA. Comparative patterns of smokeless tobacco usage among major league baseball personnel. *J Oral Pathol Med* 1989; **18**: 322–6

10 Hatsukami DK, Keenan RM, Anton DJ. Topographical features of smokeless tobacco use. *Psychopharmacology* 1988; **96**: 428–9

11 Carmella SG, Kagan SS, Kagan M *et al.* Mass spectrometric analysis of tobacco-specific nitrosamine hemoglobin adducts in snuff dippers, smokers, and nonsmokers. *Cancer Res* 1990; **50**: 5438–45

12 Holm H, Jarvis MJ, Russell MA, Feyerabend C. Nicotine intake and dependence in Swedish snuff takers. *Psychopharmacology* 1992; **108**: 507–11

13 Jansson T, Romert L, Magnusson J, Jenssen D. Genotoxicity testing of extracts of a Swedish moist oral snuff. *Mutat Res* 1991; **261**: 101–15

14 Niphadkar MP, Contractor QQ, Bhisey RA. Mutagenic activity of gastric fluid from chewers of tobacco with lime. *Carcinogenesis* 1994; **15**: 927–31

15 Johansson SL, Saidi J, Osterdahl BG, Smith RA. Promoting effect of snuff in rats initiated by 4-nitroquinoline-N-oxide or 7,12-dimethylbenz(a)anthracene. *Cancer Res* 1991; **51**: 4388–94

16 Mörnstad H, Axéll T, Sundström B. Clinical picture of snuff dipper's lesion in Swedes. *Community Dent Oral Epidemiol* 1989; **17**: 97–101

17 Ernster VL, Grady DB, Greene JC *et al.* Smokeless tobacco use and health effects among baseball players. *JAMA* 1990; **264**: 218–24

18 Livingston GK, Reed RN, Olson BL, Lockey JE. Induction of nuclear aberrations by smokeless tobacco in epithelial cells of human oral mucosa. *Environ Mol Mutagen* 1990; **15**: 136–44

19 Tolbert PE, Shy CM, Allen JW. Micronuclei and other nuclear anomalies in buccal smears: a field test in snuff users. *Am J Epidemiol* 1991; **134**: 840–50

20 Wood MW, Medina JE, Thompson GC, Houck JR, Min KW. Accumulation of the p53 tumor-suppressor gene product in oral leukoplakia. *Otolaryngol Head Neck Surg* 1994; **111**: 758–63

21 Lewin F, Rutqvist LE, Johansson H, Wennerberg J. Risk factors for larynx: case-control study of the head and neck (abstract). In: *Proceedings of the 2nd World Conference on Laryngeal Cancer.* Sydney: University of Sydney, 1994

22 Wynder EL, Hultberg S, Jacobsson F, Bross IJ. Environmental factors in cancer of the upper alimentary tract: a Swedish study with special reference to Plummer-Vinson (Paterson-Kelly) syndrome. *Cancer* 1957; **10**: 470–87

23 Winn DM, Blot WJ, Shy CM, Pickle LW, Toledo A, Fraumeni Jr JF. Snuff dipping and oral cancer among women in the southern United States. *N Engl J Med* 1981; **304**: 745–9

24 Zahm SH, Blair A, Holmes FF, Boysen CD, Robel RJ, Fraumeni Jr JF. A case-control study of soft tissue sarcoma. *Am J Epidemiol* 1989; **130**: 665–74

25 Sterling TD, Rosenbaum WL, Weinkam JJ. Analysis of the relationship between smokeless tobacco and cancer based on data from the National Mortality Followback Survey. *J Clin Epidemiol* 1992; **45**: 223–31

26 Bolinder G, Alfredsson L, Englund A, de Faire U. Smokeless tobacco use and increased cardiovascular mortality. *Am J Public Health* 1994; **84**: 399–404

27 Saranath D, Chang SE, Bhoite LT *et al*. High frequency mutation in codons 12 and 61 of *H-ras* oncogene in chewing tobacco-related human oral carcinoma in India. *Br J Cancer* 1991; **63**: 573–8

28 Kaur J, Srivastava A, Ralhan R. Overexpression of p53 protein in betel- and tobacco-related human oral dysplasia and squamous-cell carcinoma in India. *Int J Cancer* 1994; **58**: 340–5

29 Schroeder KL, Chen MS. Smokeless tobacco and blood pressure. *N Engl J Med* 1985; **312**: 919

30 Bolinder GM, Ahlborg BO, Lindell JH. Use of smokeless tobacco: blood pressure elevation and other health hazards found in a large-scale population survey. *J Intern Med* 1992: **232**: 327–34

31 Eliasson M, Lundblad D, Hägg E. Cardiovascular risk factors in young snuff-users and cigarette smokers. *J Intern Med* 1991; **230**: 17–22

32 Siegel D, Benowitz N, Ernster VL, Grady DG, Hauck WW. Smokeless tobacco, cardiovascular risk factors, and nicotine and cotinine levels in professional baseball players. *Am J Public Health* 1992; **82**: 417–21

33 Tucker LA. Use of smokeless tobacco, cigarette smoking, and hypercholesterolemia. *Am J Public Health* 1989; **79**: 1048–50

34 Eliasson M, Asplund K, Evrin PE, Lundblad D. Relationship of cigarette smoking and snuff dipping to plasma fibrinogen, fibrinolytic variables and serum insulin. The Northern Sweden MONICA study. *Atherosclerosis*: 1995: In press

35 Huhtasaari F, Asplund K, Lundberg V, Stegmayr B, Wester PO. Tobacco and myocardial infarction: is snuff less dangerous than cigarettes? *BMJ* 1992; **305**: 1252–6

36 Persson G, Hellers G, Ahlbom A. Use of oral moist snuff and inflammatory bowel disease. *Int J Epidemiol* 1993; **22**: 1101–3

Beneficial effects of nicotine and cigarette smoking: the real, the possible and the spurious

John A. Baron

Departments of Medicine, and Community and Family Medicine, Dartmouth Medical School, Hanover, New Hampshire, USA

Cigarette smoking is an established risk factor for cancer and cardiovascular disease, and is the leading cause of avoidable disease in most industrialized countries. Less well-known are possible beneficial effects, which are briefly considered in this survey.

Preliminary data suggest that there may be inverse associations of smoking with uterine fibroids and endometriosis, and protective effects on hypertensive disorders and vomiting of pregnancy are likely. Smoking has consistently been found to be inversely related to the risk of endometrial cancer, but cancers of the breast and colon seem unrelated to smoking. Inverse associations with venous thrombosis and fatality after myocardial infarction are probably not causal, but indications of benefits with regard to recurrent aphthous ulcers, ulcerative colitis, and control of body weight may well reflect a genuine benefit. Evidence is growing that cigarette smoking and nicotine may prevent or ameliorate Parkinson's disease, and could do so in Alzheimer's dementia. A variety of mechanisms for potentially beneficial effects of smoking have been proposed, but three predominate: the 'anti-estrogenic effect' of smoking; alterations in prostaglandin production; and stimulation of nicotinic cholinergic receptors in the central nervous system.

Even established inverse associations cannot be used as a rationale for cigarette smoking. These data can be used, however, to clarify mechanisms of disease, and point to productive treatment or preventive options with more narrowly-acting interventions.

It is evident from other papers in this symposium that cigarette smoking is a potent health hazard, almost certainly the leading avoidable cause of mortality and morbidity in most industrialized countries. The health burden of smoking is largely due to well-established increases in the risk of serious chronic disorders, including coronary artery disease and stroke, chronic lung disease, and many cancers[1]. Less well-known are suggestions that cigarette smoking might actually confer some beneficial effects in certain circumstances. This review surveys the conditions for which some benefits have been claimed, and considers briefly the evidence in support of these possible benefits.

©The British Council 1996

Gynecological and obstetric conditions and events

Cigarette smoking has been noted to have an 'anti-estrogenic' effect, since women who smoke cigarettes behave as though they were relatively estrogen-deficient[2,3]. This effect would be expected to have a beneficial impact on diseases and processes associated with estrogen excess, and several of the gynaecological and obstetric conditions that have been proposed to be inversely related to cigarette smoking are thought to be the consequence of estrogenic stimulation.

Uterine fibroids and endometriosis

In many regards, the presence of fibroids reflects estrogenic influences: women who are lean or postmenopausal have a lower prevalence of these tumours[4,5], although oestrogen replacement therapy has only inconsistently been related to risk[4,6]. Available data also suggest that smoking may be inversely related to the risk of having fibroids[4-6], with heavy smokers having about half the risk of never smokers, even after control for covariables such as age, body weight, and menopausal status.

Endometriosis is another disorder that seems to respond to estrogenic stimuli, and has been inversely related to cigarette smoking in several studies[7-9]. Initiation of the habit at an early age may be required for this effect, although the available data are insufficient to clarify this point.

Effects during pregnancy: nausea/vomiting and hypertensive disorders

Vomiting of pregnancy is the third oestrogen-related condition[10] that has been noted to be less common in smokers than in non-smokers[e.g. 10-13]. However, the data are not conclusive: the possibility of confounding has not been extensively considered, and adjusted relative risk estimates have not been consistently less than 1.0[14,15].

A lower incidence of hypertensive disorders of pregnancy among smokers has been regularly found. Pre-eclampsia and eclampsia have been investigated in several studies, and a 30–50% reduction in risk has been reported among smokers[e.g. 16-21]. Although early studies did not control for confounding, this has been done in the more recent investigations, with essentially no effect on the risk estimates. Smoking during the second half of pregnancy may be the most relevant exposure[18]. Gestational hypertension is also less common among smokers than among non-smokers, although the effect is somewhat less pronounced than for pre-eclampsia/eclampsia[16,18,22-24].

The mechanisms that could explain an effect of smoking on hypertensive disorders of pregnancy are not clear. Several possibilities have been proposed, including inhibition of thromboxane production, limitation of plasma volume expansion during pregnancy, and hypotensive effects of the thiocyanate contained in cigarette smoke[21].

Dysmenorrhea

One report that cigarette smokers have less dysmenorrhea compared with non-smokers[25] prompted speculation that inhibition of prostaglandin production might explain the reduced pain[26]. Other investigations, however, have reported no association, or (more commonly) increased dysmenorrhea among smokers[e.g.27–31]. Thus the data actually suggest an **increased** risk among smokers.

Down syndrome

Several studies have reported that smoking mothers have a reduced risk of delivering an infant with Down syndrome compared with non-smoking mothers[32,33]. However, in some of these investigations there was inadequate control for maternal age, and other studies reported no association, or only a weak one[34,35]. Currently, the issue remains unresolved.

Neoplasia

Tobacco and cigarette smoke are clearly rich sources of carcinogens, and greatly increase the risk of cancer at virtually all anatomic sites having direct contact with tobacco or tobacco smoke, as well as at some sites that lack such contact[36]. There have also been suggestions that smoking might have an inverse relationship with the risk of neoplasia at some locations that do not have smoke contact — where direct carcinogenesis is not an issue, and where other effects of smoking might play a protective role.

Fibrocystic breast disease and breast cancer

Fibrocystic breast disorders are a heterogenous group of processes in the breast that appear to be responsive to ovarian hormones[37]. Several studies have suggested a lower risk among smokers, especially among currently smoking postmenopausal women[6,38,39]. The data are not consistent, however, and in other analyses no association was found[40].

A few investigations have suggested that cigarette smoking may be inversely related to the risk of breast cancer[41]. These were largely case-control studies, and subsequent investigations have reported no association or even a small increase in risk[2,42,43]. Apparently, the original reports were chance findings, or possibility the result of biasing factors in the studies themselves[44]. The considerable data available on the topic indicate that there is no substantial association, either overall, or among premenopausal or postmenopausal women considered separately[2,42,43].

Endometrial cancer

Endometrial cancer is the only malignancy that has repeatedly been shown to be inversely related to cigarette smoking[2,45]. The association is stronger among postmenopausal women, and seems to be absent in former smokers. A dose–response pattern has been found in several studies, with a relative risk of 0.5 or less among heavy smokers in comparison to never smokers. The association remains even after control for the effects of lower body weight and earlier age at menopause in smokers. In some studies, but by no means all, the association was particularly marked among women taking exogenous estrogens[2,45], a pattern consistent with the hypothesis that smoking may be acting to alter the metabolism of oral estrogens.

Colorectal cancer

Some reports have suggested that cigarette smoking may be inversely related to the risk of colorectal cancer[e.g.46,47] — in particular colon cancer among women[47]. However, other epidemiological studies have not confirmed this association[48,49], or have reported an increased risk among long-term smokers[50]. Although the possibility of an increased risk remains controversial, the available data clearly do not suggest that smoking has an inverse association with colon cancer.

One investigation reported that among patients with ulcerative colitis, cigarette smokers had a lower risk of bowel cancer than non-smokers[51]. The association was not statistically significant, however, and the issue has not been extensively studied; the suggestion remains a speculative one.

Cardiovascular Disease

Survival after myocardial infarction

Several studies have suggested that cigarette smokers have a lower case fatality after myocardial infarction than non-smokers (reviewed in[52]), with a reduction in fatality of 40% or greater in some reports. Several explanations for this association have been advanced, including differences between smokers and non-smokers in the types of arterial lesions that precipitate infarction, the beneficial effects of the smoking cessation enforced by hospital admission, and confounding by other prognostic factors. The last possibility is almost certainly part of the effect; strong associations between smoking and potent prognostic factors have been demonstrated[e.g.52], and in many reports on the topic the control for confounding — even by age — has been inadequate.

Venous thrombosis

In the 1970s, there were several reports that smokers had a lower risk of deep venous thrombosis after hospital admission for myocardial infarction[53-55], gynaecological surgery[56] or other reasons[57]. The relative risks that can be computed from the data presented are strikingly low: 0.25 or lower. Some later data were similar[58], but most of these studies did not consider possible confounding, even by age. Other, often more formal, studies have failed to confirm the finding[59-63]. However, these negative studies have focussed on slightly different clinical events than the ones that suggested a benefit. All were conducted among women, and none focussed on in-patient venous thrombosis, as did the earlier reports. The literature regarding pulmonary embolism provides some clarification: there are no suggestions of protective effect of smoking, although the data are not extensive[64-66].

In many ways, an anti-thrombotic effect of cigarette smoking would seem implausible; smoking is generally thought to exert a pro-coagulant effect through increased fibrinogen levels, reduced fibrinolysis, and probably through platelet activation[67-69]. However, there is *in vitro* evidence that nicotine and cotinine can inhibit synthesis of prostaglandins, including thromboxane, a potent proaggregatory prostanoid[68,70-72]. These direct prostaglandin-inhibiting effects of nicotine could conceivably lead to a decreased risk of thrombosis, although it remains to be demonstrated that these *in vitro* effects have *in vivo* clinical significance.

Inflammatory and immunological disorders

Cigarette smoking has been shown to affect several measures of immune functioning, including those of T-cell functioning and antibody response[73]. The usual concern is that this immune suppression may lead to a susceptibility to infections, although it is conceivable that the impairment could be beneficial for immunologically-mediated disorders.

Aphthous ulcers

An inverse association between cigarette smoking or smokeless tobacco use and the risk of recurrent aphthous ulceration of the oral mucosa has been reported in several studies, though not in all[e.g.74–77]. Some investigators have also published case reports noting a worsening of the ulcers after smoking cessation, with relief after resumption[e.g.78,79]. It has been proposed that the increased oral keratinization associated with tobacco use could explain the inverse association; the possible efficacy of nicotine chewing gum suggests that nicotine is an active moiety[80].

One study reported that another oral disorder, herpes labialis, is less prevalent in tobacco users than in non-users[81]. However, the differences were small, confounding was not considered, and the finding seems not to have been confirmed.

Ulcerative colitis

An inverse association between cigarette smoking and ulcerative colitis has been repeatedly documented. The relationship is complex, since current smokers have a markedly reduced risk relative to never smokers (as low as 0.4 or lower), but former smokers have, if anything, an increased risk[82,83].

Reports of the amelioration of ulcerative colitis symptoms by smoking[e.g.84] or nicotine administration[85,86] led to formal trials of transdermal nicotine. The pattern of response resembles that of cortico-steroid therapy: transdermal nicotine aided the treatment of patients in relapse[87], but a somewhat less intense nicotine regimen was ineffective in prolonging remission[88].

Thus there is considerable evidence that smoking—and nicotine in particular–has a beneficial effect in ulcerative colitis. The effect remains unexplained, although several mechanisms have been proposed, including changes in bowel mucus or prostaglandins, immune suppression, and other effects in the bowel[89].

Extrinsic allergic alveolitis

Smoking seems clearly to be inversely related to extrinsic allergic alveolitis (farmers' lung, pigeon breeders' lung), a chronic immunologi-cally-mediated lung disorder. Several studies have noted an inverse association of cigarette smoking with the clinical syndrome[90–93], and numerous investigations have documented that serum antibodies to the antigens associated with the disorder are reduced[e.g.73,91,92,94–96]. The suppressive effect of smoking on antibody levels may be reversible, since former smokers seem to have antibody levels intermediate between current smokers and never smokers[91,92,94,96].

Hay fever and atopy

A lower prevalence of hay fever was noted among smokers in one study[97] and other reports have found that smokers are less likely to react to skin prick testing with common seasonal antigens[98–100]. Reactions to occupational antigens, however, seem to be enhanced[100]. Aside from the need for clarification of these discrepant findings, there is at least one issue that hampers interpretation of these data: it is not clear if smoking impairs the immune response related to atopy, or if atopic individuals have difficulty even starting to smoke because of allergic symptoms.

Sarcoidosis

Several case-control studies have reported an inverse association between smoking and the risk of sarcoidosis[101–106]. However, the control groups used by many of these investigations do not closely correspond to the cases, and it is possible that selection bias may have distorted the findings. Also, some negative reports have been published[90,107], and the possibility of confounding by social class has explicitly been raised[107]. The association thus remains uncertain, although the effects of smoking on lymphocyte populations make it plausible[104,105].

Acne

One study with clinic cases and general population controls reported an inverse association between cigarette smoking and severe acne[108], a finding which has been ascribed to impaired inflammatory responses in smokers[100]. No other evidence regarding the association seems to be available.

Metabolic effects

Body weight

An inverse association between cigarette smoking and body weight is well established[109,110]. The weight difference between smokers and non-smokers appears to be larger at older ages, and is most marked for moderate smokers. Cessation of smoking is associated with weight gain, a factor which impedes smoking control efforts. Animal data support the association[110].

Several possible mechanisms have been advanced for the effects of smoking on body weight[109,110]. Laboratory data and prospective studies suggest that smoking is associated with a decreased caloric intake, although cross-sectional investigations tend not to confirm this[110]. In any case, the effect of smoking is not completely explained by differences in energy intake or physical activity; several studies have shown that cigarette smokers have a higher metabolic rate than non-smokers[111-113]. Most of the weight-reducing effects of smoking seem to be due to nicotine, although there are suggestions of a behavioral component as well[113].

Central nervous system functioning

There are several reasons why an effect of cigarette smoking or nicotine administration might plausibly have an effect on the functioning of the central nervous system. Nicotinic cholinergic receptors are widespread in the brain[114] and chronic nicotine administration increases their density[115]. Presumably as a consequence of stimulation of these receptors, nicotine leads to the release of several neurotransmittors with potentially important functional consequences[116].

Motor system disorders: Parkinsonism and Tourette's syndrome

An inverse association between cigarette smoking and Parkinson's disease is well established[117-119]. Numerous epidemiological studies have confirmed the apparent protective effect, with ever smokers having a relative risk about 0.5 in comparison to never smokers. Although most of the research has involved case-control study of prevalent cases, cohort investigations and mortality studies have also supported these findings. In aggregate, the data overcome most biases that have been proposed to explain the association[117-119]. However, the possibility that individuals destined to be at high risk for Parkinson's disease may have an aversion to smoking has not been completely excluded.

The inverse relationship of smoking with Parkinson's disease may well reflect a genuine biological effect. Some animal studies, but not all, have shown that cigarette smoke or nicotine can ameliorate experimental Parkinsonism[120-123]. Also, some case reports and a more formal double-blind trial have suggested a benefit of nicotine administration in patients with Parkinsonism[124,125]. Moreover, nicotine appears to effect several disorders of the extrapyramidal motor system in addition to Parkinson's disease: smoking or nicotine can reduce drug-induced Parkinsonism, ameliorate Tourette's syndrome, and worsen neuroleptic tardive dyskinesia, effects that all point to effects on dopaminergic motor systems[119,126].

Alzheimer's disease

The epidemiological data regarding a possible inverse association between cigarette smoking and Alzheimer's dementia is fairly consistent; most studies have reported an inverse association, although there are reports to the contrary[118,127,128]. As for Parkinson's disease, much of the research involves case-control studies with prevalent cases. Alzheimer's epidemiology is complicated by the difficulties of distinguishing Alzheimer's dementia from other dementing illnesses, and (in case-control research) by the need for surrogate respondents. However, the plausibility of a protective effect of smoking on Alzheimer's disease is supported by reports that short-term nicotine administration may provide modest improvements in measures of mental functioning in patients with Alzheimer's disease[129,130].

Mental functioning

In addition to effects in Parkinson's disease and Alzheimer's dementia, smoking may also effect mental performance in non-diseased individuals. Research conducted among smokers has shown that cigarette smoking (or nicotine administration) has several benefits, including modest improvements in vigilance and information processing, facilitation of some motor responses, and perhaps enhancement of memory[131-133]. Also, smoking or nicotine clearly ameliorates the mild deterioration in mental functioning associated with nicotine withdrawal. The effects of nicotine in non-smokers are not as clear. The use of smokers in much of the cognitive research has necessarily involved individuals with chronic nicotine exposure; this may well alter acute affects through tolerance or receptor changes, or through the distortions associated with nicotine withdrawal. Nonetheless, there are certainly data suggesting benefits of nicotine in non-smokers with regard to performance and information processing[131-135]. Consistent with these findings, experimental studies in animals have suggested that nicotine may improve learning and memory, although some investigations showed evidence of nicotine-associated impairments[132].

Mechanisms

A variety of mechanisms have been invoked to explain the relationships described. Several of the proposed beneficial effects involve disorders that are associated with estrogen-excess (endometrial cancer, uterine fibroids, endometriosis, fibrocystic breast disease). The anti-estrogenic effect is itself unexplained, but may involve induced changes in the metabolism of estrogens, direct toxic effects on ovarian follicles, or interference with pituitary regulation of sex hormone systems[2]. A second group of possible benefits involves the effects of smoking on central nervous system neurotransmitter systems[116]. These effects could plausibly explain associations of smoking with Parkinson's disease, Alzheimer's dementia, and mental functioning. Third, there are clear indications that smoking can alter prostaglandin pathways, and suppress at least some aspects of immunological functioning[68,73]. These effects could underlie the associations of smoking with ulcerative colitis, farmers' lung and hypertensive disorders of pregnancy.

These benefits are not without their costs, however. The antiestrogenic effect of smoking may at least partially explain the association of smoking with an increased risk of osteoporotic fractures[2] and the central nervous system effects of nicotine clearly underlie tobacco dependence[109]. Inhibition of prostaglandin synthesis is thought to play a role in the effects of smoking on vascular disease[67].

Conclusions

Some of the proposed beneficial effects of smoking are not real. The effect of smoking on survival after myocardial infarction is at least partly artifactual, and smokers do not have a lower risk of dysmenorrhoea, colorectal cancer, and breast cancer as has been suggested. For effects on Down syndrome and venous thrombosis, the available data are not sufficient for conclusions to be drawn, and the association remains speculative; no convincing mechanisms have been proposed. For other conditions, possible benefits are more plausible, but remain unproven. These include functionally important improvements in mental functioning and Alzheimer's dementia, and inverse associations with sarcoidosis. Finally, the available evidence is very suggestive of a genuine benefit with regard to endometrial cancer, aphthous ulcers, ulcerative colitis, external allergic alveolitis, Parkinson's disease, and control of body weight.

These associations can hardly be used to justify cigarette smoking; its adverse effects are simply too overwhelming. However, these data do provide insight into the mechanisms of several diseases, and suggest avenues for treatments and preventive measures that are likely to be far safer than cigarette smoking.

References

1 Bartecchi CE, MacKenzie TD, Schrier RW. The human costs of tobacco use. *N Engl J Med* 1994; **330**: 907–12

2 Baron JA, La Vecchia C, Levi F. The antiestrogenic effect of cigarette smoking in women. *Am J Obstet Gynecol* 1990; **162**: 502–14

3 Wald N, Baron J. *Smoking and Hormone-Related Disorders*. Oxford: Oxford University Press, 1990

4 Ross RK, Pike MC, Vessey MP *et al*. Risk factors for uterine fibroids: reduced risk associated with oral contraceptives. *BMJ* 1986; **293**: 359–61

5 Parazzini F, La Vecchia C, Negri E *et al*. Epidemiologic characteristics of women with uterine fibroids: a case-control study. *Obstet Gynecol* 1988; **72**: 853–7

6 Wyshak G, Frisch RE, Albright NL *et al*. Lower prevalence of benign diseases of the breast and benign tumours of the reproductive system among former college athletes compared to non-athletes. *Br J. Cancer* 1986; **54**: 841–5

7 Cramer DW, Wilson E, Stillman RJ *et al*. The relation of endometriosis to menstrual characteristics, smoking, and exercise. *JAMA* 1986; **255**: 1904–8

8 Darrow SL, Vena JE, Batt RE *et al*. Menstrual cycle characteristics and the risk of endometriosis. *Epidemiology* 1993; **4**: 135–42

9 Matorras R, Ramon O, Rodiquez F *et al*. Epidemiology of endometriosis in infertile women. *Fertil Steril* 1995; **63**: 34–8

10 Depue RH, Bernstein L, Ross RK *et al*. Hyperemesis gravidarum in relation to estradiol levels, pregnancy outcome, and other maternal factors: a seroepidemiologic study. *Am J Obstet Gynecol* 1987; **156**: 1137–41

11 Little RE, Hook EB. Maternal alcohol and tobacco consumption and their association with nausea and vomiting during pregnancy. *Acta Obstet Gynecol Scand* 1979; **58**: 15–17

12 Vellacott ID, Cooke EJA, James CE. Nausea and vomiting in early pregnancy. *Int J Gynecol Obstet* 1988; **27**: 57–62

13 Meyer LC, Peacock JL, Bland JM, Anderson HR. Symptoms and health problems in pregnancy: their association with social factors, smoking, alcohol, caffeine and attitude to pregnancy. *J Paediatr Perinat Epidemiol* 1994; **8**: 145–55

14 Klebanoff MA, Koslowe PA, Kaslow R, Rhoads GG. Epidemiology of vomiting in early pregnancy. *Obstet Gynecol* 1985; **66**: 612–16

15 Weigel MM, Weigel RM. The association of reproductive history, demographic factors, and alcohol and tobacco consumption with the risk of developing nausea and vomiting in early pregnancy. *Am J Epidemiol* 1988; **127**: 562–70

16 Underwood PB, Kesler KF, O'Lane JM, Callagan DA. Parental smoking empirically related to pregnancy outcome. *Obstet Gynec* 1967; **29**: 1–8

17 Duffus GM, MacGillivray I. The incidence of pre-eclamptic toxaemia in smokers and non-smokers. *Lancet* 1968; i: 994–5

18 Marcoux S, Brisson J, Fabia J. The effect of cigarette smoking on the risk of preeclampsia and gestational hypertension. *Am J Epidemiol* 1989; **130**: 950–7

19 Eskenazi B, Fenster L, Sidney S. A multivariate analysis of risk factors for preeclampsia. *JAMA* 1991; **266**: 237–41

20 Klonoff-Cohen H, Edelstein S, Savitz D. Cigarette smoking and preeclampsia. *Obstet Gynecol* 1993; **81**: 541–4

21 Spinillo A, Capuzzo E, Egbe TO, Nicola S, Piazzi G, Baltaro F. Cigarette smoking in pregnancy and risk of pre-eclampsia. *J Human Hypertension* 1994; **8**: 771–5

22 Andrews J, McGarry JM. A community study of smoking in pregnancy. *J Obstet Gynaecol Br Commonwealth* 1972; **79**: 1057–73

23 Hoff C, Wertel W, Blackburn WR *et al*. Trend associations of smoking with maternal, fetal, and neonatal morbidity. *Obstet Gynecol* 1986; **689**: 317

24 Savitz DA, Zhang J. Pregnancy-induced hypertension in North Carolina, 1988 and 1989. *Am J Public Health* 1992; **82**:675–9

25 Andersch B, Milsom I. An epidemiologic study of young women with dysmenorrhea. *Am J Obstet Gynecol* 1982; **144**: 655–60

26 Backon J. Negative correlation of cigarette smoking and dysmenorrhea: reduced prostaglandin synthesis due to beta-endorphin, nicotine, or acrolein antagonism. *Med Hypotheses* 1989; **28**: 213–14

27 Wood C, Larsen L, Williams R. Social and psychological factors in relation to premenstrual tension and menstrual pain. *Aust NZ J Obstet Gynaecol* 1979; **19**: 111–15

28 Sloss EM, Frerichs RR. Smoking and menstrual disorders. *Int J Epidemiol* 1983; **12**: 107–9

29 Brown S, Vessey M, Stratton I. The influence of method of contraception and cigarette smoking on menstrual patterns. *Br J Obstet Gynaecol* 1988; **95**: 905–10

30 Sundell G, Milsom I, Andersch B. Factors influencing the prevalence and severity of dysmenorrhoea in young women. *Br J Obstet Gynaecol* 1990; **97**: 588–94

31 Parazzini F, Tozzi L, Mezzopane R *et al*. Cigarette smoking, alcohol consumption, and risk of primary dysmenorrhea. *Epidemiology* 1994; **5**: 469–72

32 Hook EB, Cross PK. Cigarette smoking and Down syndrome. *Am J Hum Genet* 1985; **37**: 1216–24

33 Hook EB, Cross PK. Maternal cigarette smoking Down syndrome in live births, and infant race. *Am J Hum Genet* 1988; **42**: 482–9

34 Cuckle HS, Alberman E, Wald JN *et al*. Maternal smoking habits and Down's syndrome. *Prenat Diagn* 1990; **10**: 561–7

35 Van Den Eeden SK, Karagas MR, Daling JR, Vaughan TL. A case-control study of maternal smoking and congenital malformations. *Paediatr Perinat Epidemiol* 1990; **4**: 147–55

36 US Department of Health and Human Services. *The Health Consequences of Smoking: 25 Years of Progress*. A report of the Surgeon General. US Department of Health and Human Services, Public Health Service, Office on Smoking and Health. DHHS Publication no. (CDC) 89-8411, 1989

37 Vorherr H. Fibrocystic breast disease: pathophysiology, pathomorphology, clinical picture, and management. *Am J Obstet Gynecol* 1986; **154**: 161–79

38 Berkowitz G, Canny PF, Vivolsi VA *et al*. Cigarette smoking and benign breast disease. *J Epidemiol Community Health* 1985; **39**: 308–13

39 Pastides H, Najjar MA, Kelsey JL. Estrogen replacement therapy and fibrocystic breast disease. *Am J Prev Med* 1987; **3**: 282–6

40 Rohan TE, Baron JA. Cigarette smoking and benign breast disease. In: Wald N, Baron J. eds. *Smoking and Hormone-Related Disorders*. Oxford: Oxford University Press, 1990: pp 72–80

41 Baron JA. Smoking and estrogen-related disease. *Am J Epidemiol* 1984; **119**: 9–22

42 MacMahon B. Cigarette smoking and cancer of the breast. In: Wald N, Baron J. eds. *Smoking and Hormone-Related Disorders*. Oxford: Oxford University Press, 1990: pp 154–66

43 Palmer JR, Rosenberg L. Cigarette smoking and the risk of breast cancer. *Epidemiol Rev* 1993; **15**: 145–56

44 Meara J. McPherson K, Roberts M *et al*. Alcohol, cigarette smoking and breast cancer. *Br J Cancer* 1989; **60**: 70–3

45 Weiss NS. Cigarette smoking and the incidence of endometrial cancer. In: Wald N, Baron J. eds. *Smoking and Hormone-Related Disorders*. Oxford: Oxford University Press, 1990: pp 145–53

46 Garland C, Barrett-Connor E, Rossof AH. Dietary vitamin D and calcium and risk of colorectal cancer: a 19-year prospective study in men. *Lancet* 1985; **i**: 307–9

47 Sandler RS, Sandler DP, Comstock GW *et al*. Cigarette smoking and the risk of colorectal cancer in women. *J Natl Cancer Inst* 1988; **80**: 1329–33

48 Baron JA, Sandler RS. Cigarette smoking and cancer of the large bowel. In: Wald N, Baron J. eds. *Smoking and Hormone-Related Disorders*. Oxford: Oxford University Press, 1990: pp 167–80

49 Baron JA, Gerhardsson de Verdier M, Ekbom A. Coffee, tea, tobacco, and cancer of the large bowel. *Cancer Epidemiol Biomarkers Prevention* 1994; **3**: 565–70

50 Giovanucci E, Rimm EB, Stampfer MJ *et al*. A prospective study of cigarette smoking and risk of colorectal adenoma and colorectal cancer in U.S. men. *J Natl Cancer Inst* 1994; **86**: 183–91

51 Pinczowski D, Ekbom A, Baron J *et al*. Risk factors for colorectal cancer in patients with ulcerative colitis: a case-control study. *Gastroenterology* 1994; **107**: 117–20

52 Barbash GI, White HD, Modan M *et al*. Significance of smoking in patients receiving thrombolytic therapy for acute myocardial infarction. *Circulation* 1993; **87**: 53–8

53 Handley AJ, Teather D. Influence of smoking on deep vein thrombosis after myocardial infarction. *BMJ* 1974; **3**: 230–1

54 Emerson PA, Marks P. Preventing thromboembolism after myocardial infarction: effect of low-dose heparin or smoking *BMJ* 1977; **1**: 18–20

55 Marks P, Emerson PA. Increased incidence of deep vein thrombosis after myocardial infarction in non-smokers. *BMJ* 1977; **3**: 232–4

56 Clayton JK, Anderson JA, McNicol GP. Effect of cigarette smoking on subsequent postoperative thromboembolic disease in gynaecological patients. *BMJ* 1978; **2**: 402

57 Prescott RJ, Jones DRB, Vasilescu CV *et al*. Smoking and risk factors in deep vein thrombosis. *Thrombos Haemostas* 1978; **40**: 128–33

58 Crandon AJ, Koutts J. Incidence of post-operative deep vein thrombosis in gynaecological oncology. *Aust NZ J Obstet Gynaecol* 1983; **23**: 216–19

59 Vessey MP, Doll R. Investigation of relation between use of oral contraceptives and thromboembolic disease. A further report. *BMJ* 1969; **2**: 651–7

60 Stolley PD, Tonascia JA, Tockman MS *et al*. Thrombosis with low-estrogen oral contraceptives. *XXX* 1975; **102**: 197–208

61 Hayes MJ, Morris GK, Hampton JR. Lack of effect of bed rest and cigarette smoking on development of deep venous thrombosis after myocardial infarction. *Br Heart J* 1976; **38**: 981–3

62 Petitti DB, Wingerd J, Pellegrin F, Ramcharan S. Oral contraceptives, smoking, and other factors in relation to risk of venous thromboembolic disease. *Am J Epidemiol* 1978; **108**: 480–5

63 Vandenbroucke JP, Koster T, Briet E *et al*. Increased risk of venous thrombosis in oral-contraceptive users who are carriers of factor V Leiden mutation. *Lancet* 1994; **344**: 1453–7

64 Arthes FG. An epidemiologic survey of hospitalized cases of venous thrombosis and pulmonary embolism in young women. *Milbank Q* 1972; **50** (Suppl 2): 233–43

65 Samkoff JS, Comstock GW. Epidemiology of pulmonary embolism: mortality in a general population. *Am J Epidemiol* 1981; **114**: 488–96

66 Goldhaber SZ, Savage DD, Garrison RJ *et al*. Risk factors for pulmonary embolism. The Framingham Study. *Am J Med* 1983; **74**: 1023–8

67 FitzGerald GA, Oates JA, Nowak J. Cigarette smoking and hemostatic function. *Am Heart J* 1988; **115**: 267–71

68 Jeremy JY, Mikhailidis DP. Smoking and vascular prostanoids: relevance to the pathogenesis of atheroma and thrombosis. *J Smoking-Related Dis* 1990; **1**: 59–69

69 Benowitz NL, FitzGerald GA, Wilson M, Zhang Q. Nicotine effects on eicosanoid formation and hemostasis function: comparison of transdermal nicotine and cigarette smoking. *J Am Coll Cardiol* 1993; **22**: 1159–67

70 Ylikorkala O, Viinikka L, Lehtovirta P. Effect of nicotine on fetal prostacyclin and thromboxane in humans. *Obstet Gynecol* 1985; **66**: 102–5

71 Goerig M, Ullrich V, Schettler G *et al*. A new role for nicotine: selective inhibition of thromboxane formation by direct interaction with thromboxane synthase in human promyelocytic leukaemia cells differentiating into macrophages. *Clin Invest* 1992; **70**: 239–43

72 Saareks V, Riutta A, Much I *et al*. Nicotine and cotinine modulate eicosanoid production in human leukocytes and platelet rich plasma. *Eur J Pharmacol* 1993; **248**: 345–9

73 Holt PG. Immune and inflammatory function in cigarette smokers. *Thorax* 1987; **42**: 241–9

74 Shapiro S, Olson DL, Chellemi SJ. The association between smoking and aphthous ulcers. *Oral Surg Oral Med Oral Pathol* 1970; **30**: 624–30

75 Axell T, Henricsson V. Association between recurrent aphthous ulcers and tobacco habits. *Scand J Dent Res* 1985; **93**: 239–42

76 Zain RB, Razak IA. Association between cigarette smoking and prevalence of oral mucosal lesions among Malaysian army personnel. *Community Dent Oral Epidemiol* 1989; **17**: 148–9

77 Grady D, Ernster VL, Stillman L, Greenspan J. Smokeless tobacco use prevent aphthous stomatitis. *Oral Surg Oral Med Oral Pathol* 1992; **74**: 463–5

78 Bookman R. Relief of canker sores on resumption of cigarette smoking. *California Med* 1960; **93**: 235

79   Sallay K, Banoczy J. Remarks on the possibilities of the simultaneous occurrence of hyperkeratosis of the mucous membranes and recurrent aphthae. *Oral Surg* 1968; **25**: 171–5

80   Bittoun R. Recurrent aphthous ulcers and nicotine. *Med J Aust* 1991; **154**: 471–2

81   Axell T, Liedholm R. Occurrence of recurrent herpes labialis in an adult Swedish population. *Acta Odontol Scand* 1990; **48**: 119–23

82   Calkins BM. A meta-analysis of the role of smoking in inflammatory bowel disease. *Dig Dis Sci* 1989; **34**: 1841–54

83   Thomas GAO, Rhodes J. Relationship between smoking, nicotine and ulcerative colitis. In: Clarke PBS, Quik M, Adlkofer F, Thurau K. eds. *Effects of Nicotine on Biological Systems II.* Basel: Birkhauser, 1995: pp 287–91

84   De Castella H. Non-smoking: a feature of ulcerative colitis (letter). *BMJ* 1982; **284**: 1706

85   Roberts CJ, Diggle R. Non-smoking: a feature of ulcerative colitis. *BMJ* 1982; **285**: 440

86   Lashner BA, Hanauer SB, Silverstein MD. Testing nicotine gum for ulcerative colitis patients. *Dig Dis Sci* 1990; **35**: 827–32

87   Pullan RD, Rhodes J, Ganesh S et al. Transdermal nicotine for active ulcerative colitis. *N Engl J Med* 1994; **330**: 811–15

88   Thomas GAO, Rhodes J, Mani V et al. Transdermal nicotine as maintenance therapy for ulcerative colitis. *N Engl J Med* 1995; **332**: 988–92

89   Rhodes J, Thomas GAO. Smoking: good or bad for inflammatory bowel disease? *Gastroenterology* 1994; **106**: 807–10

90   Warren CPW. Extrinsic allergic alveolitis: a disease commoner in non-smokers. *Thorax* 1977; **32**: 567–9

91   Gruchow HW, Hoffmann RG, Marx JJ et al. Precipitating antibodies to farmer's lung antigens in a Wisconsin farming population. *Am Rev Respir Dis* 1981; **124**: 411–15

92   McSharry C, Banham SW, Boyd G. Effect of cigarette smoking on the antibody response to inhaled antigens and the prevalence of extrinsic allergic alveolitis among pigeon breeders. *Clin Allergy* 1985; **15**: 487–94

93   Terho EO, Husman K, Vohlonen I. Prevalence and incidence of chronic bronchitis and farmer's lung with respect to age, sex, atopy, and smoking. *Eur J Resp Dis* 1987; **152** (Suppl): 1–28

94   Cormier Y, Belanger J, Durand P. Factors influencing the development of serum precipitins to farmer's lung antigen in Quebec dairy farmers. *Thorax* 1985; **40**: 138–42

95   Terho EO, Husman K, Vohlonen I, Mantyjarvi RA. Serum precipitins against microbes in mouldy hay with respect to age, sex, atopy, and smoking of farmers. *Eur J Resp Dis* 1987; **152** (Suppl): 115–21

96   Kusaka H, Homma Y, Ogasawara H et al. Five-year follow-up of *Micropolyspora faeni* antibody in smoking and nonsmoking farmers. *Am Rev Respir Dis* 1989; **140**: 695–9

97   Bakke P, Gulsvik A, Eide GE. Hay fever, eczema and urticaria in southwest Norway. *Allergy* 1990; **45**: 515–22

98   Burrows B, Lebowitz MD, Barbee RA. Respiratory disorders and allergy skin-test reactions. *Ann Intern Med* 1976; **84**: 134–9

99   Oryszczyn M-P, Annesi I, Neukirch F et al. Relationships of total IgE level, skin prick test response, and smoking habits. *Ann Allergy* 1991; **67**: 355–8

100 Mills CM, Hill SA, Marks R. Altered inflammatory responses in smokers. *BMJ* 1993; **307**: 911

101 Comstock GW, Keltz H, Sencer DJ. Clay eating and sarcoidosis. *Am Rev Respir Dis* 1961; **84** (Suppl): 130–4

102 Terris M, Chaves AD. An epidemiologic study of sarcoidosis. *Am Rev Respir Dis* 1966; **94**: 50–5

103 Douglas JG, Middleton WG, Gaddie J et al. Sarcoidosis: a disorder commoner in non-smokers? *Thorax* 1986; **41**: 787–91

104 Harf RA, Ethevenaux C, Gleize J et al. Reduced prevalence of smokers in sarcoidosis. *Ann NY Acad Sci* 1986; **145**: 625–31

105 Hance AJ, Basset F, Aumon G et al. Smoking and interstitial lung disease. *Ann NY Acad Sci* 1986; **145**: 643–56

106 Revsbech P. Is sarcoidosis related to exposure to pets or the housing conditions? A case-referent study. *Sarcoidosis* 1992; **9**: 101–3

107 Bresnitz EA, Stolley PD, Israel HL, Soper K. Possible risk factors for sarcoidosis. *Ann NY Acad Sci* 1986; **145**: 632–42

108 Mills CM, Peters TJ, Finlay AY. Does smoking influence acne? *Clin Exp Dermatol* 1993; **18**: 100–1

109 US Department of Health and Human Services. *The Health Consequences of Smoking: Nicotine Addiction*. A report of the Surgeon General. US Department of Health and Human Services, Public Health Service, Office on Smoking and Health. DHHS Publication no (CDC) 88-8406, 1988

110 Grunberg NE. The inverse relationship between tobacco use and body weight. In: Kozlowski LT, Annis HM, Cappel HD *et al*. eds. *Research Advances in Alcohol and Drug Problems*, vol 10. New York: Plenum, 1990: pp 273–315

111 Hofstetter A, Schutz Y, Jéquier E, Wahren J. Increased 24-hour energy expenditure in cigarette smokers. *N Engl J Med* 1986; **314**: 79–82

112 Perkins KA, Epstein LH, Marks BL, Stiller RL, Jacob RG. The effect of nicotine on energy expenditure during light physical activity. *N Engl J Med* 1989; **320**: 898–903

113 Perkins KA, Epstein LH, Marks BL, Stiller RL, Jacob RG. The effects of nicotine on resting metabolic rate in cigarette smokers. *Am J Clin Nutr* 1989; **50**: 545–50

114 Leutje CW, Patrick J, Seguela P. Nicotine receptors in the mammalian brain. *FASEB J* 1990; **4**: 2753–60

115 Benwell MEM, Balfour DJK, Anderson JM. Evidence that tobacco smoking increases the density of (–)-[^{3}H]-nicotine binding sites in human brain. *J Neurochem* 1988; **50**: 1243–7

116 Rowell RP. Current concepts on the effects of nicotine on neurotransmitter release in the central nervous system. In: Martin WR, VanLoon GR, Iwamoto ET, Davis L. eds. *Tobacco Smoking and Nicotine*. New York: Plenum, 1987: pp 191–208

117 Baron JA. Cigarette smoking and Parkinson's disease. *Neurology* 1986; **36**: 1490–6

118 Graves AB, Mortimer, JA. Does smoking reduce the risk of Parkinson's and Alzheimer's diseases? *J Smoking Related Dis* 1994; **5** (Suppl 1): 79–90

119 Baron JA. The epidemiology of cigarette smoking and Parkinson's disease. In: Clarke PBS, Quik M, Adlkofer F, Thurau K. eds. *Effects of Nicotine on Biological Systems II*. Basel: Birkhauser, 1995: pp 313–19

120 Janson AM, Meana JJ, Goiny M, Herrera-Marschitz M, Chronic nicotine treatment counteracts the decrease in extracellular neostriatal dopamine induced by a unilateral transection at the mesodiencephalic junction in rats: a microdialysis study. *Neurosci Lett* 1991; **134**: 88–92

121 Sershen H, Hashim A, Lajtha A. Behavioral and biochemical effects of nicotine in an MPTP-induced mouse model of Parkinson's disease. *Pharmacol Biochem Behav* 1987; **28**: 299–303

122 Carr LA, Rowell PP. Attenuation of 1-methyl-4-phenyl-1,2,3,6-tetrahydropyridine-induced neurotoxicity by tobacco smoke. *Neuropharmacology* 1990; **29**: 311–14

123 Shahi GS, Das N, Moochhala SM. 1-methyl-4-phenyl-1,2,3,6-tetrahydropyridine-induced neurotoxicity: partial protection against striato-nigral dopamine depletion in C%&BL/6J mice by cigarette smoke exposure and by β-naphthoflavone-pretreatment. *Neurosci Lett* 1991; **127**: 247–50

124 Ishikawa A, Miyatake T. Effects of smoking in patients with early-onset Parkinson's disease. *J Neurol Sci* 1993; **117**: 28–32

125 Fagerström KO, Pomerleau O, Giordani B, Stelson F. Nicotine may relieve symptoms of Parkinson's disease. *Psychopharmacology* 1994; **116**: 117–19

126 Newhouse PA, Hughes JR. The role of nicotine and nicotinic mechanisms in neuropsychiatric disease. *Br J Addict* 1991; **86**: 521–6

127 Graves AB, van Duijn CM, Chandra V *et al*. Alcohol and tobacco consumption as risk factors for Alzheimer's disease: a collaborative re-analysis of case-control studies. *Int J Epidemiol* 1991; **20** (Suppl 2): S48–S57

128 Breteler MMB, Claus JJ, van Duijn CM, Launer LJ, Hofman A. Epidemiology of Alzheimer's disease. *Epidemiol Rev* 1992; **14**: 59–82

129 Jones GMM, Sahakian BJ, Levy R *et al*. Effects of acute subcutaneous nicotine on attention, information processing and short-term memory in Alzheimer's disease. *Psychopharmacology* 1992; **108**: 485–94

130   Newhouse PA, Potter A, Piasecki M *et al*. Nicotinic modulation of cognitive functioning in humans. In: Clarke PBS, Quik M, Adlkofer F, Thurau K. eds. *Effects of Nicotine on Biological Systems II*. Basel: Birkhauser, 1995: pp 345–51

131   Wesnes K, Warburton DM. Smoking nicotine and human performance. *Pharmacol Ther* 1983; **21**: 189–208

132   Levin ED. Nicotinic systems and cognitive function. *Psychopharmacology* 1992; **108**: 417–31

133   Heishman SJ, Taylor RC, Henningfield JE. Nicotine and smoking: a review of effects on human performance. *Exp Clin Psychopharmacol* 1994; **2**: 345–95

134   Wesnes K. Nicotine increases mental efficiency: but how? In: Martin WR, Van Loon GR, Iwamoto ET, Davis L. eds. *Tobacco Smoking and Nicotine: A Neurobiological Approach*. New York: Plenum, 1987: pp 63–79

135   Le Houezec J, Halliday R, Benowitz NL, Callaway E, Naylor H, Herzig K. A low dose of subcutaneous nicotine improves information processing in non-smokers. *Psychopharmacology* 1994; **114**: 628–34

Women and smoking

Amanda Amos

Department of Public Health Sciences, University of Edinburgh, Edinburgh, UK

Smoking kills over half a million women each year and is the most important preventable cause of female premature death in several developed countries. However, in many countries, cigarette smoking still tends to be regarded as a mainly male problem. This paper explores the reasons why more attention needs to be paid to issues around smoking and women, even in countries which currently have low levels of female cigarette smoking. The article includes an overview of current patterns and trends of smoking among women, and the factors which influence smoking uptake and cessation in women compared to men. The experience of countries with the longest history of widespread female smoking is used to identify some of the key challenges facing developed and developing countries. Tobacco companies have identified women as a key target group, therefore particular attention is given to the ways in which they have attempted to reach women through advertising and other marketing strategies. It is concluded that in order to halt and ultimately reverse the tobacco epidemic among women, tobacco control policies need to encompass both gender-specific and gender-sensitive approaches. Examples are given of the types of action that are needed in relation to research, public policy and legislation, and education.

Smoking kills over half a million women around the world each year and this number is increasing rapidly[1]. It is estimated that between 1950 and 2000, 10 million women will have died from their smoking habit. In several developed countries, such as the USA and the UK, cigarette smoking is now the single most important preventable cause of premature death in women, accounting for at least a third of all deaths in women aged 35 to 69[1]. Yet, despite these figures, smoking is still regarded in many countries as being a mainly male problem. This is due primarily to two main reasons.

1. Cigarette smoking prevalence among women in many countries, particularly developing countries, is still low compared to men.
2. Because of the time lag between smoking becoming a widespread habit and the emergence of tobacco-related health problems, no country has yet experienced the full impact of smoking on women's health.

©The British Council 1996

This article aims to explore each of these reasons and consider why more attention needs to be paid to issues around smoking among women, both in terms of research and action, even in countries where female smoking prevalence is currently low. In particular, it will examine the assumption that the factors which influence smoking uptake and cessation are the same for men and women and thus tobacco control programmes can be gender-neutral. Drawing on a review of the current patterns and trends of smoking among women across the world, it will be argued that unless more action is taken to address the reasons why, on the one hand, women take up smoking and, on the other, find it hard to quit, the smoking epidemic will continue to spread rapidly. The experience of countries with the longest history of widespread female smoking will be used to identify key issues in both developed and developing countries, and to argue the case for gender-specific and gender-sensitive approaches to tobacco control.

This paper will focus primarily on cigarette smoking, as this is the most prevalent form of tobacco use among women. However, when relevant, reference will be made to other types of traditional tobacco use which are common in certain parts of the world.

Patterns and trends — the growing epidemic

A cursory look at the data on cigarette smoking prevalence in different countries might suggest that there are no consistent patterns or trends among women (Table 1). Prevalence rates vary from as much as 58% in Nepal and over a third in European countries, such as Denmark and Poland, to barely detectable levels in many African countries, such as the Ivory Coast and Guinea[2]. Somewhat more consistent is the finding that cigarette smoking rates are higher among men than women. However, there is some considerable variation between countries, with equal or nearly equal rates in the USA and UK, but several-fold differences in countries such as China, where less than 6% of women are daily smokers compared to 56% of men (Table 1).

However, a more detailed examination of the data reveals that these variations are not random but rather reflect different stages of the smoking epidemic in each country. Recently, a four stage model has been developed, based on evidence from countries with the longest history of cigarette smoking, which describes the typical evolution of cigarette smoking and subsequent mortality in a country (Fig. 1)[3]. While the exact picture in each country will vary to some degree, countries can be characterised as falling into one of four different evolutionary stages:

Table 1 Prevalence of cigarette smoking among women in selected countries (Source: see[2], apart from China data[38])

Region	Prevalence (%)	Date of survey
Americas		
Bolivia	38	1986
Brazil	33	1990
Guyana	4	—
Honduras	11	1988
Jamaica	27	1988
Trinidad and Tobago	5	1986–89
USA	26	1990
Europe		
Denmark	45	1988
France	30	1991
Germany	27	1988
Poland	35	1989
Portugal	12	1988
Spain	28	1988
UK	28	1992
Africa		
Ivory Coast	1	1981
Guinea	1	1981
Nigeria	10	1990
Swaziland	7	1989
Zambia	4–7	1984
Eastern Mediterranean		
Bahrain	20	1985
Egypt	2	1981
Sudan	19	1986
Tunisia	6	1984
South East Asia		
India	0–67[a]	—
Indonesia	10	1990
Nepal	58	1991
Thailand	4	1988
Western Pacific		
Australia	27	1986–89
China	5[b]	1991
Japan	14	1990
Malaysia	5	1990
New Zealand	26	1986–89
Singapore	2	1988

[a]Depends on area surveyed; [b]Small study of rural women

Stage 1   (e.g. many developing countries mainly in sub-Saharan Africa). Male prevalence rates less than 15% but increasing rapidly, female prevalence less than 5%. Health consequences not yet apparent.

Stage 2   (e.g. China, Japan, several countries in Asia, Latin America and North Africa). Male prevalence rates rising rapidly to 50–80% with few

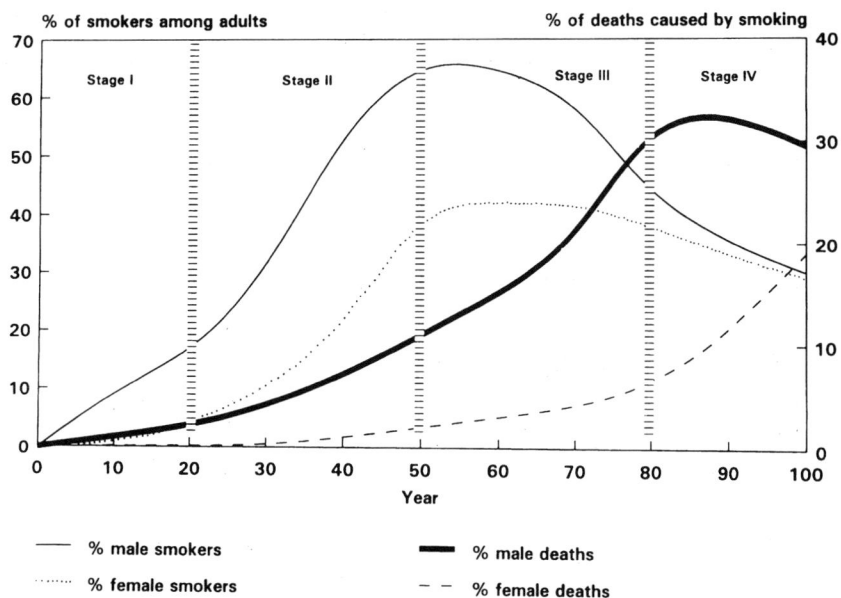

Fig. 1 A model of the cigarette epidemic (Source: see[1])

ex-smokers. Female rates lagging 10–20 years behind but increasing. Male smoking related death rates starting to increase.

Stage 3 (e.g. Eastern and Southern Europe). Male prevalence starting to decline, reaching around 40%. Female prevalence peaks and plateaus at a lower rate than among men, and starts to decline by the end of this stage.

Stage 4 (e.g. USA, UK, Canada, Western Europe). Smoking declining slowly in both sexes. Male mortality from smoking peaks as female deaths begin to rise rapidly.

This model has several important features which need to be taken into account when considering women and smoking.

1. Women generally take up cigarette smoking as a widespread habit later than men. This is mainly due to socio-cultural factors, such as it not being socially acceptable for women to be seen smoking in public, religious attitudes, and women generally being less affluent than men and, therefore, unable to afford cigarettes. However, this model indicates that countries with low female smoking rates should not be complacent. If cigarette smoking is increasing among men, then it is likely to increase among women in the future. Indeed, while in countries such as the UK and the USA there was a 20–30 year lag between smoking becoming a widespread habit in men and women, more recent evidence from several Stage 2 and 3 countries suggests

this lag may now be much shorter, particularly where there is aggressive promotion of cigarettes to women and/or there are rapid changes in women's socio-economic position. Thus the challenge for countries in Stages 1 and 2 is to take action now to counter the factors that encourage smoking among women, especially girls and young women.

2. Even in countries where smoking among women is increasing (Stages 2 and 3), there may be little awareness or concern about this trend, as female rates of smoking will be considerably lower than those in men, and the health consequences for women will not have started to emerge. However, the model predicts that unless effective action is taken, smoking is likely to continue to increase amongst women and thus become a major cause of death. This is not inevitable. For example, the approach adopted by Singapore in the 1970s, when it was at the beginning of Stage 2, showed that implementing a strong and comprehensive tobacco control policy can reverse this trend and the progression from Stages 1 to 2. Female smoking declined from 9.5% in 1978 to 3% in 1992[3].

3. The women who are most likely to start smoking in large numbers are those who are most affluent, well educated and live in urban areas (Stages 1 and 2). For example, in Costa Rica, a survey found that 24% of affluent, urban women were smokers compared with only 10% of poor, rural women[4]. Similarly, a survey carried out in Spain in 1989 showed that 21% of women smoked compared to 52% of men, and the largest number of female smokers was in the highest socio-economic group. 52% of upper class compared to 12% of working class women smoked[5]. However, more advantaged women are also more likely to show the first declines in smoking, reflecting both lower rates of uptake and higher cessation rates (Stages 3 and 4). Thus, in countries where smoking is declining, smoking is increasingly associated with disadvantage. In these countries, the typical female smoker has a limited education, a low status job or is unemployed, is on a low income and experiences high levels of other aspects of deprivation. For example, in the UK in 1992, 13% of women in socio-economic group 1 smoked compared to 35% in socio-economic group 6, and whereas 62% of professional women who had ever smoked had given up, only 36% of unskilled manual women had succeeded in quitting[6]. Also, in many countries, the highest smoking rates are found among disadvantaged ethnic minorities. For example, in Canada in 1989, 77% of Inuit women were smokers[7] and in New Zealand Maori women smoke more than white women and have one of the highest smoking rates among women in the world[2].

4. Because there is a time lag between the widespread uptake of smoking and the health effects, even countries with the longest history of female

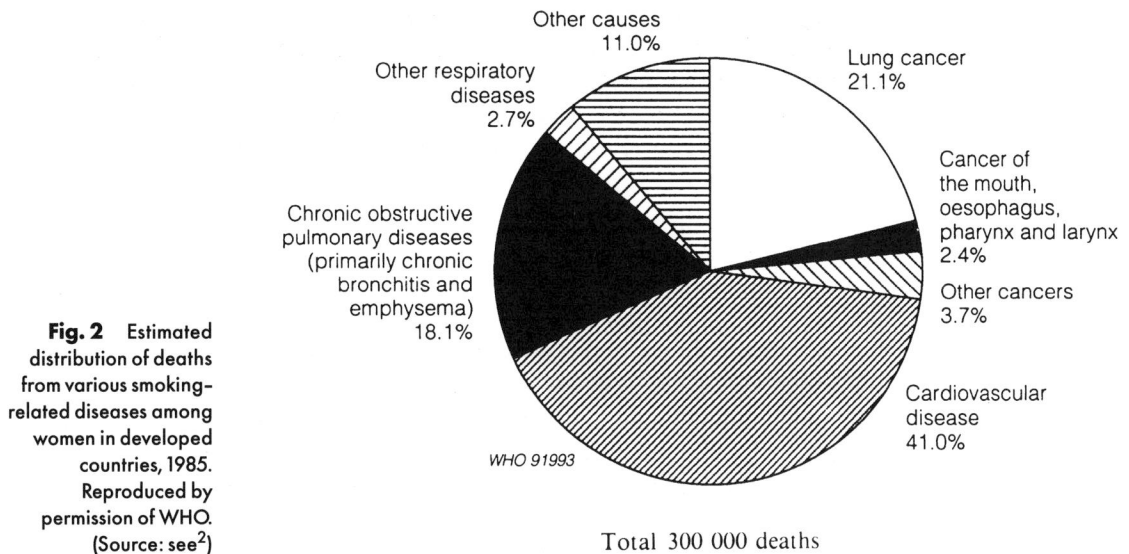

Fig. 2 Estimated distribution of deaths from various smoking-related diseases among women in developed countries, 1985. Reproduced by permission of WHO. (Source: see[2])

Other causes
11.0%

Other respiratory diseases
2.7%

Chronic obstructive pulmonary diseases (primarily chronic bronchitis and emphysema)
18.1%

Lung cancer
21.1%

Cancer of the mouth, oesophagus, pharynx and larynx
2.4%

Other cancers
3.7%

Cardiovascular disease
41.0%

WHO 91993

Total 300 000 deaths

smoking have not yet experienced smoking's full impact on women's health. Because men in developed countries were the first to smoke cigarettes in large numbers, most of the epidemiological research has been carried out on these male populations. Thus, our understanding of the true impact of smoking on women's health in developed and developing countries is limited. There is now, however, strong evidence which indicates that where women have smoked cigarettes regularly for several decades, the percentage of female deaths which are attributable to tobacco is now approaching the male figure[1]. It is estimated that, among women in developed countries who have smoked regularly throughout their adult lives, tobacco will cause at least half, and perhaps substantially more, of all deaths in middle age. Countries which have recently seen a big increase in smoking amongst young women, (Stages 2 and 3) such as France, Spain and Poland, will experience a large increase in female mortality early in the next century.

Thus it is clear that whatever the stage of the smoking epidemic within a country, action is urgently needed to halt its progression, for there is now no doubt that smoking among women causes the same diseases as are found among men (Fig. 2). The main tobacco killers in both sexes are cancers, especially lung cancer, heart disease and chronic bronchitis. But smoking also affects women's health in ways which are specific to them. Research in developed countries[2] has found that women who smoke: (i) have a 10-times higher risk of heart disease and an increased risk of stroke if they also use oral contraceptives; (ii) have a 2-fold associated higher risk of cervical cancer; and (iii) experience detrimental affects on their reproductive health, including dysmenorrhoea, reduced fertility and an earlier menopause. Women who smoke during pregnancy also increase by a quarter their risk of miscarriage and by a third the risk of the infant's perinatal death; they are twice as likely to have premature labour and 3-times more likely to have a low birth weight baby[8] (see also Charlton in this issue). In those developing countries, where the health of mother and baby is already jeopardised through poverty and malnutrition, the effects of smoking are likely to have an even greater impact on birth weight and perinatal mortality. In Chile, for example, it is estimated that 10% of non-accidental perinatal deaths are attributable to smoking[9].

In developing countries with high levels of traditional tobacco use among women, such as chewing or smoking with the lit end of the chutta inside the mouth, tobacco use is associated with high levels of oral cancer (see also Pershagen in this issue). For example, the highest reported rate of mouth cancer in the world is among women in Bangalore, India[2]. Indeed it is estimated that tobacco use causes around one in five of all cancers in women in India[10].

Why women smoke

The reasons why people start to smoke and quit smoking, are considered in depth in other articles in this issue. However, in order to develop effective tobacco control strategies for women, it is important to consider what is known about the extent to which the factors which influence smoking uptake and cessation differ between men and women. This section will look at some of the main findings from research which has explored these issues. Most of these studies have been carried out in developed countries which have the longest history of female cigarette smoking, and thus our understanding is somewhat limited. However, many of the issues raised are also likely to be relevant to women in developing countries (see also Mackay and Crofton in this issue).

Starting the habit

A recent WHO study of 10 European countries indicated that over a third of girls have tried smoking by the age of 13 and this increased to around 60% among 15-year-olds[11]. The initiation of smoking in girls, as in boys, is heavily influenced by social pressures and psychological needs including: environmental influences, school and peer influences, personal factors, and knowledge, attitudes and beliefs about smoking[12].

Creating the market The tobacco industry is dependent on a mass market. As smokers die or quit they are keen to recruit new young smokers to maintain their profits, particularly in new markets such as developing countries and Eastern Europe. The art of marketing is to tailor a product to appeal to specific target groups by altering its price, availability and image through packaging, advertising and promotions. Over the past few years the tobacco industry has targeted women by[13-15]:

- Promoting brands through advertisements and sponsorship using images and messages which promote smoking as being glamorous, sophisticated, romantic, sexy, healthy, sporty, fun, relaxing, liberated, rebellious and, last, but not least, slimming.
- Producing 'women only' brands, such as Virginia Slims, Kim, Charm & Eve, and other types of cigarettes which are likely to appeal to women.
- Advertising in women's magazines to reach large numbers of women and discourage reporting about the health risks—magazines that are dependent on tobacco revenues are less likely to cover the health hazards and to take anti-smoking advertisements[16,17].

The tobacco industry argues that cigarette advertisements do not encourage smoking but simply affect brand choice. Yet research in developed countries shows that children can identify the brands of edited cigarette advertisements and their awareness of cigarette brands is a strong predictor of future smoking[18]. Young teenagers who smoke are more appreciative of cigarette advertising than non-smokers; and the most heavily advertised brands are more often bought by teenagers than adult smokers[19,20].

Many developing countries have few limitations on tobacco promotion and therefore their influence on girls, who are likely to be less knowledgeable about the harmful effects of smoking, may be even more powerful. Cigarette advertising in developing countries, at present, tends to be directed at the general public, but there is evidence that women are becoming special targets. In Hong Kong, where less than 1% of young women smoke, Philip Morris launched a major campaign to promote the Virginia Slims brand—a clear attempt to create a market among young women[21]. In India, an attempt has also been made to launch a 'women only' brand. However, where widespread restrictions on tobacco promotion have been introduced, there has been an immediate fall in smoking prevalence among young people, especially girls[22].

How smoking is portrayed in the media more generally also affects the way in which young people view the habit. Glamorous models, female personalities, teenage pop idols and film stars all feature in magazines, TV soaps, plays and films which depict smoking as being part and parcel of their success. These images reach many different audiences around the world and, particularly in developing countries, may create aspirational images of western life which are both unrealistic and harmful to their audiences' health. In South Asia, for example, concerts by Madonna and Paula Abdul have been sponsored by tobacco companies.

The social setting   Adolescents are more likely to take up smoking if their parents smoke or have permissive attitudes towards smoking. In developed countries, girls, in particular, appear to be influenced by their parents' smoking habits and attitudes, although this decreases as they get older[12]. The situation is much the same in developing countries and countries where religious and cultural mores are applied more strictly to girls than boys[22]. While this pattern also holds in some ethnic communities within developed countries, this may change as girls become assimilated into the dominant culture. In countries where cigarette smoking is comparatively new among women, it is the more affluent professional women who adopt the habit first[23]. This may be due to the more liberated environment in which they live and work, their relative affluence and their urban environment which exposes them to tobacco advertisements and makes cigarettes more accessible.

First cigarettes are usually smoked with friends and having a best friend who smokes is a strong predictor of whether a young person will become a smoker, though this may be more important among boys than girls[24]. Adolescent smokers are also more likely to be underachievers at school with low academic goals. In the US, the narrowing gap in smoking rates between men and women in the 1980s was due, in part, to increasing initiation rates among less educated women. Women without a college education were over twice as likely to take up smoking as those who went to college[12].

Personal factors   Many young people in developed countries experiment with drugs, such as tobacco, in an attempt to achieve the image of maturity, sophistication, attractiveness, sociability or femininity to which they aspire. Of particular importance to girls are concerns about weight and self confidence. In western countries, where the media promote an image of female attractiveness which equates being thin with desirability, weight control and dieting are major obsessions among adolescent girls[25]. This concern has been picked up and used in advertisements for certain cigarette brands aimed at women which associate smoking with slimness and glamour [26].

Research has repeatedly found that girls with low self-esteem are more likely to take up smoking. Adolescents who feel that they have a lot of control over their health and life are less likely to become smokers than those who feel they have little control[27]. Using smoking to bolster self-confidence stems from the widespread belief that smoking can help calm nerves, control moods and alleviate stress — all important concerns during adolescence. By showing attractive young women with handsome male partners or socialising with successful and confident people, tobacco advertisements exploit young people's insecurities, and sell the idea that these desirable qualities are theirs if they smoke. There is also evidence that girls feel more dependent on cigarettes compared to boys smoking similar amounts, and imagine that they would find giving up more difficult[28].

Knowledge and attitudes Whether a girl becomes a smoker also depends on her knowledge about the health risks, whether she feels that these are personally relevant, and whether they outweigh the perceived benefits of smoking. In many developed countries, school health education programmes have been effective in increasing young people's knowledge about the health effects of smoking, increasing their awareness of influences such as advertising and social pressure, and developing their personal confidence, self-esteem and social skills to resist smoking. However, it is not clear whether they ultimately reduce smoking or simply delay its onset[12]. Since girls are more likely to believe that smoking helps them deal with stressful situations, developing their self-esteem and competency to solve problems without resorting to smoking, is likely to be an important strategy. In developing countries, girls' knowledge about smoking and health is likely to be limited due to the lack of systematic health education programmes and structural barriers, such as widespread rural populations, and high levels of illiteracy. Educational programmes are urgently needed to counteract the increasing promotional activities of tobacco companies.

Why women stay hooked

Putting up a smoke screen As public awareness about the health effects of tobacco has grown, tobacco companies have responded in many countries by increasing the amount and variety of tobacco products and promotions that are targeted specifically at women in an attempt to allay health fears[15,26]. These include cigarettes which are lower in tar, lower in nicotine or are mentholated. Many women have changed to low tar cigarettes believing that this reduces their health risks. There is, however, little medical evidence to support this view[29]. Low tar cigarettes do not lower heart disease risk. Some studies have found that people who switch to lower nicotine cigarettes compensate by inhaling more deeply or smoking more often.

The pressures on women In countries with the longest history of widespread female smoking, smoking is now most common among those on low incomes, who have low status jobs or are unemployed, are single parents or divorced, have low levels of academic achievement and are from under-privileged ethnic groups. One reason why these women continue this habit at such cost to their health and finances is their belief that cigarettes help them cope[25,30].

A woman on a low income, tied to the home, bringing up small children on her own may smoke to deal with her feelings of stress or to calm her nerves. Although recognising that it may ultimately damage her own health, she may feel that smoking may be less damaging to her children than 'letting off steam' some other way. Similarly, women at home may structure their day with cigarettes, providing excuses for breaks and refuelling. Women in low status, repetitive and insecure jobs may also smoke to break the monotony or deal with the frustration and irritation of the work. Many women on low incomes, with little time to themselves, see cigarettes as their only luxury — the only thing they do for themselves. In reality, smoking probably does little to relieve stress, calm nerves or reduce feelings of anger, but, as long as women believe that it does, they are unlikely to feel that they can cope competently without cigarettes.

Gaining weight — the price of giving up?   Many women in developed countries also believe that smoking helps control their weight and quitting leads to weight gain[31,32]. Studies have shown a weight gain around 5–10 lbs after giving up smoking among some women. Even so, the disadvantages, in terms of health, of a small weight gain are more than offset by the health benefits. Whether the weight gain is due to changes in metabolic rate, changes in palate or eating more is not certain. It is clear, however, that, for many women, a small weight gain is a high cost to pay in terms of their self-image and this needs to be recognised. There is a need to develop ways of helping women to quit without gaining weight.

An addictive habit   As a young woman starts to smoke regularly, her body gets used to regular nicotine doses and she becomes physiologically dependent. She develops a pattern of daily smoking which, together with having partners and friends who smoke, and her beliefs about smoking, act to reinforce this dependency. In order to quit, women need help and support to overcome short term physiological withdrawal, and to break behavioural patterns that may have developed over many years.

Kicking the habit

Cessation clinics in developed countries have tended to show that women are less successful than men in quitting[33] but this cannot be generalised to all women since the vast majority who quit successfully do so independently. That women in the USA, UK and Australia are now giving up at about the same rate as men also refutes this notion[34]. These figures, however, do not show the relative success of men and women in maintaining their non-smoking, for example do women have to make more attempts at quitting than men before they are successful? The differences in cessation rates between different groups of women are, however, indisputable. Disadvantaged women are less likely to give up smoking than more affluent women[2,25,30]. If these women are to be empowered to take control of their lives, it will be necessary to adopt strategies that address not only their smoking but also the social and economic circumstances that reinforce their habit[35].

In countries where smoking is on the decline, it has been generally found that most women want to give up. Many have attempted to quit at least once and most make several attempts before they are successful. Confidence in the ability to quit and the desire and resolve to succeed are of crucial importance[36]. Most people go through a process that involves precontemplation, contemplation, action, maintenance and relapse. Cessation programmes that address all stages of the giving up process are likely to be the most effective. Individual programmes will be given added support if they are backed up by measures aimed at changing the social and environmental factors which make giving up easier and cater for the needs of non-smokers.

Issues for action

Smoking is a complex issue and controlling its spread requires a comprehensive approach. However, it seems that while similar factors influence smoking among men and women there appear to be some important differences, often relating to girls' and women's own social worlds, which need to be taken into account. In order to achieve the overall aim of helping young women to resist pressures to start smoking and to help women who smoke to quit, tobacco control strategies need to be both gender-sensitive and specific. These strategies need to encompass three areas of action.

Research

Many countries lack comprehensive and reliable data about women and smoking, such as patterns and trends of smoking and smoking-related diseases. Such information is crucial for the effective development, implementation and evaluation of programmes. Countries also need to develop their understanding of women's reasons for smoking and quitting, and, in particular, be aware of factors which might encourage smoking, such as cigarette promotion aimed at girls and women. Further research is needed to explore more fully the role that smoking plays in women's daily lives and how health promotion can help women develop alternative ways of dealing with the factors that keep them smoking.

Public policy and legislation

The aim is to create a social, economic and political climate which promotes non-smoking as the norm and reduces countries' economic dependence on the production, manufacture and sale of tobacco. This will require combined action at the international, national, and community levels. It is essential that women become more visible and that the issue of women and smoking is placed high on the health agenda. This will be facilitated through exchanging information, expertise and research. The establishment of the International Network of Women Against Tobacco (INWAT) provides an important channel for communication and support for people concerned about this issue. INWAT, for example, was instrumental in setting up the *First International Conference on Women and Smoking* in 1992, and has since published newsletters including a special issue of World Smoking and Health 'Herstories'[37]. While formal and informal networks such as INWAT have helped give a greater visibility to women and smoking, many countries have yet to acknowledge the potential seriousness of this issue. It is, therefore, important that health professionals and other concerned people seize the initiative and raise the awareness of policy makers, key professionals and the public about the threat that smoking poses to women's health.

Education and support

It is essential that girls and women have the knowledge, attitudes and skills to help them make informed decisions about smoking. To be effective, programmes need to be culturally appropriate, relevant to girls' and women's needs at different points in their lives, and related to the stage of the smoking epidemic in the country. Each country needs to design a strategy which meets their circumstances and takes into account gender differences. There is a need for gender-sensitive and gender-specific programmes. For example, women tend to have more contact with the health service thus creating considerable opportunities for health education. This is particularly important in relation to smoking and pregnancy. Health education should also form an integral part of school education. However, education should not just be restricted to health and educational services. In many developing countries, girls have only limited access to schooling, and in Stages 3–4 countries, smoking is more common among academic under-achievers and those whose who are disenchanted with school. It is, therefore, important to involve organisations and networks which reach women in different ways, such as youth organisations, community groups and networks, women's organisations, workplaces, and the media including women's magazines, radio and TV. Many of these agencies have been largely silent on this issue.

Conclusion

Smoking is a major cause of ill-health and premature death among women in many countries and this is increasing rapidly. Even in countries where smoking is still low among women, many women's lives are already negatively affected by smoking, for example through their husbands' spending scarce resources on cigarettes, their constant exposure to second-hand smoke and, increasingly, having to cope with a spouse's death from smoking. While religious and cultural attitudes, often combined with low economic status, have kept female smoking levels low in many countries, history shows that unless strong, comprehensive tobacco control policies are implemented, female smoking prevalence will increase. The tobacco industry has identified women as a key target group around the world. Countries with newly opened markets, such as China and Eastern Europe, or which have no restrictions on tobacco promotion, are particularly vulnerable to mass targeting by the tobacco industry. Also vulnerable are girls and women in countries undergoing fast urbanisation or industrialisation, where tobacco promotion attempts to associate smoking with aspirational images such as affluence, sophistication, modernity and success. Firm action needs to be taken now to halt and ultimately reverse this epidemic.

Acknowledgements

I would like to thank Yvonne Bostock for her many valuable comments and discussions and Morag Leitch for typing the manuscript.

For further information about INWAT contact Deborah McLellan at the American Public Health Association, 1015 Fifteenth Street NW, Washington DC, USA.

References

1 Peto R, Lopez AD, Boreham J, Thun M, Heath C. *Mortality from Smoking in Developed Countries 1950–2000*. Oxford: Oxford University Press, 1994

2 Chollat-Traquet C. *Women and Tobacco*. Geneva: World Health Organization, 1992

3 Lopez AD, Collishaw NE, Piha T. A descriptive model of the cigarette epidemic in developed countries. *Tobacco Control* 1994; **3**: 242–7

4 Rosero-Bixby L, Oberle MW. Tobacco use in Costa Rican women. *Ciencias Sociales* 1987; **35**: 95–102

5 Ministerio de Sanidad y Consumo. *Estudio de los estilos de vida de la población adulta espanola*. Madrid: Ministerio de Sanidad y Consumo, Dirección General de Salud Publica, 1992

6 OPCS. *General Household Survey 1992*. London: HMSO, 1994

7 Miller W, Peterson J. *Tobacco Use by Youth in the Canadian Arctic, 1989*. Ottawa: Health and Welfare Canada and Ministry of Health NWT, 1989

8 Royal College of Physicians. *Smoking and the Young*. London: Royal College of Physicians, 1992

9 US Surgeon General. *Reducing the Health Consequences of Smoking: 25 Years of Progress*. Maryland: Department of Health and Human Services, 1989

10 Stanley K, Stjernsward J. Lung cancer in developing countries. In: Hansen HH, ed. *Basic Clinical Concepts of Lung Cancer*. Boston: Kluyer Academic, 1989

11 Currie C, Todd J, Thomson C. *Health behaviours of Scottish school children. Report 4. The cross-national perspective: Scotland compared to other European countries and Canada*. Edinburgh: Health Education Board for Scotland, 1994

12 US Department of Health and Human Services. *Preventing tobacco use among young people: a report of the Surgeon General*. Atlanta: US Department of Health and Human Services, 1994

13 Ernster VL. Mixed messages for women: a social history of cigarette smoking and advertising. *NY State J Med* 1985; **316**: 725–32

14 Amos A, Bostock Y. *Putting women in the picture: cigarette advertising policy and coverage of smoking and health in women's magazines in Europe*. London: BMA, 1992

15 Amos A. How women are targeted by the tobacco industry. *World Health Forum* 1990; **11**, 416–22

16 Warner KE, Goldenhar LM, McLaughlin CG. Cigarette advertising and magazine coverage of the hazards of smoking: a statistical analysis. *N Engl J Med* 1992; **326**: 305–9

17 Penna RM. The essence of censorship. *Tobacco Control* 1994; **3**: 104–5

18 Aitken PP. *Children and cigarette advertising: Smoke-Free Europe 8*. WHO: Copenhagen, 1988

19 Difranza JR, Richards JW, Paulman PM *et al*. RJR Nabisco's cartoon camel promotes Camel cigarettes to children. *J Am Med Assoc* 1991; **266**: 3149–53

20 Hastings GB, Ryan H, Teer P, Mackintosh AM. Cigarette advertising and children's smoking: why Reg was withdrawn. *BMJ* 1994; **309**: 933–6

21 Chapman S. *Pushing smoke-tobacco advertising and promotion: Smoke-Free Europe 8*. Copenhagen: WHO, 1988

22 Waldron I, Bratelli G, Carriker L. Sung W-C, Vogeli C, Waldman E. Gender differences in tobacco use in Africa, Asia, the Pacific and Latin America. *Soc Sci Med* 1988; **27**: 1269–75

23 Mackay J. Women and tobacco, the scale of the problem: developing countries. *Proceedings of the First International Conference on Women and Smoking*. Belfast: Ulster Cancer Foundation/ Health Promotion Agency for Northern Ireland, 1993; p 32–34

24 Charlton A, Blair V. Predicting the onset of smoking in boys and girls. *Soc Sci Med* 1989; **29**: 813–18

25 Greaves L. *Background Paper: women and tobacco (1987) and Update (1990)*. Ottawa: Health and Welfare Canada, 1990
26 Davis RM. Current trends in cigarette advertising and marketing. *N Engl J Med* 1987; **316:** 725–32
27 Nutbeam D, Mendoza R. Newman R. *Planning for a smoke-free generation: Smoke-Free Europe 6*. Copenhagen: WHO, 1988
28 Goddard E. *Why Children Start Smoking*. London: HMSO, 1990
29 Palmer JR, Rosenberg L, Shapiro S. 'Low yield' cigarettes and the risk of nonfatal myocardial infarction in women. *N Engl J Med* 1989; **320:** 1569–73
30 Graham H. *When Life's a Drag — Women, Smoking and Disadvantage*. London: HMSO, 1993
31 Rigotti NA. Cigarette smoking and weight gain. *N Engl J Med* 1989; **320:** 931–3
32 Batten L. Respecting sameness and difference: taking account of gender in research and smoking. *Tobacco Control* 1993; **2:** 185–6
33 US Department of Health and Human Services. *The health consequences of smoking: nicotine addiction. A report of the Surgeon General*. Maryland: CDC, 1988
34 Jarvis MJ. Gender differences in smoking cessation: real or myth? *Tobacco Control* 1994; **3:** 324–8
35 Crossan E, Amos A. *Under a Cloud — Women, Low Income and Smoking*. Edinburgh: Health Education Board for Scotland, 1994
36 Marsh A, Matheson J. *Smoking Attitudes and Behaviour*. London: HMSO, 1983
37 Greaves L, Jordan J, MeLellan D (eds) Herstories. *World Smoking Health* 1994; **19:** 2
38 Niv S, He X, Wang G. A national smoking prevalence and health consequence survey in China in 1991. *Proceedings of the 9th World Conference on Tobacco and Health*. Paris: CNIT, 1994; 29

Children and smoking: the family circle

Anne Charlton

Cancer Research Campaign, Education and Child Studies Research Group, School of Epidemiology and Health Sciences, University of Manchester, Manchester, UK

Children's and adults' smoking can form a 'family circle'. Young women and their male partners who are less well-educated and less affluent are most likely to smoke during the woman's pregnancy. The harmful effects on the fetus, including low birth weight and increased risk of respiratory diseases, are carried forward into childhood. The frequent minor ailments can cause absence from school, falling behind with school work and perhaps under-achievement. Children of mothers who smoked during pregnancy are likely to have smaller stature which can also affect self-esteem.

Passive smoking in the home exacerbates these effects and adds others.

The child, therefore, can become disenchanted with school and reject its norms and is then at increased risk of becoming a smoker. These young smokers are most likely to leave school early, to start families early and to smoke during pregnancy, thus continuing the 'family circle' or 'cycle of deprivation'. Practical action is needed.

The issue of children and smoking is, both socially and healthwise, a circular one. Children's smoking behaviour is related to that of adults, especially to that of their parents; their health is affected by adult smoking; their behaviour is affected by their health; this is then carried forward into adulthood to affect the next generation of children. It is perhaps best described as 'a cycle of deprivation', or 'family circle', although the smokers involved would be unlikely to interpret it in that way. The circular nature of the problem makes it difficult to choose the best point at which to start an overview. However, a brief consideration of the historical aspects is helpful in setting the scene and leads naturally from the adult smoking to children's smoking.

The development of smoking

Rogers and Shoemaker developed a theory of the communication of innovations, which can be applied to both the rise and fall of cigarette smoking in a country (Fig. 1)[1]. The behaviour, in this case cigarette smoking, is started by a few innovators and is then taken up by a

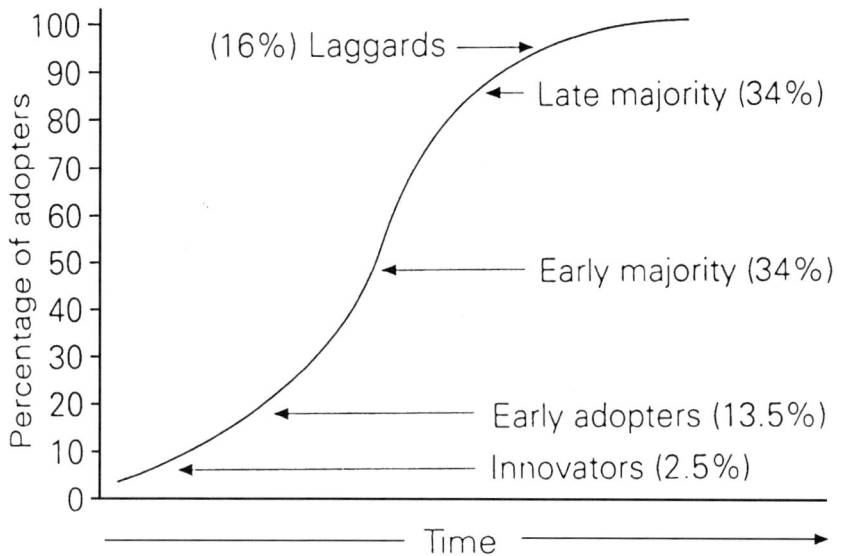

Fig. 1 The S-shaped diffusion curve and adopter categories (after Rogers and Shoemaker, 1971: reproduced by kind permission from: Tones K, Tilford S, Robinson Y. *Health Education: Effectiveness, Efficiency and Equity.* **Chapman and Hall, 1994; p. 85)**

relatively small group of 'early adopters'. This group has a particular set of characteristics, including being better-educated, more affluent, perhaps in a decision-making role and socially advantaged. In most countries, and Britain was no exception when cigarette smoking was introduced, this group is usually the men in the higher socio-economic groups. It can be seen worldwide and is especially clearly illustrated in the US Surgeon General's report[2]. After the behaviour has become established in these early adopters, it is taken up by the 'early majority' and the 'late majority', which, for reasons of social status and norms, is usually the 'blue collar' men. In many countries, it is still socially unacceptable for women to smoke, but, as western habits spread by means of the media to these areas and emancipation of women is seen as desirable, women next become the adopters of cigarette smoking followed by the girls, both groups following the diffusion of innovations curve (Fig. 2). This situation is developing in China at present[3]. In Britain, the USA, Canada, Australia, New Zealand and other industrialised countries, this process has gone the whole way. However, the reverse process also begins when the first messages about health risks are received. Again it is the 'white collar' men who act on it first and become non-smokers as they did in response to the report by the Royal College of Physicians in 1962[4-6]. Boys, women and finally girls develop their own 'diffusion of innovations' curve in adopting non-smoking. Men and women with lower socio-economic status are again mainly in the 'late majority' group in taking up a new behaviour. Therefore in most westernised countries the point has been reached where smoking prevalence has fallen

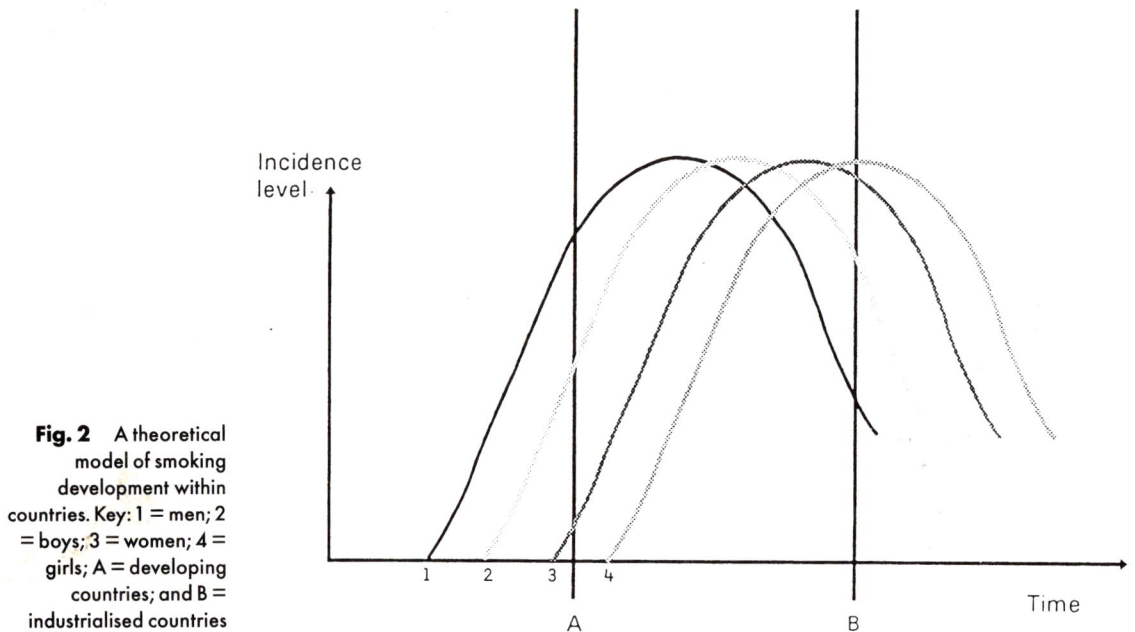

Fig. 2 A theoretical model of smoking development within countries. Key: 1 = men; 2 = boys; 3 = women; 4 = girls; A = developing countries; and B = industrialised countries

considerably among the more affluent men and women and also among boys. Girls' smoking prevalence is still high, as it is among the less affluent or less well-educated men and women[6] (Table 1).

Children's smoking prevalence, especially that of girls, is, therefore, a major problem in Britain. What has happened, since the first national survey of children's smoking in 1966[7], is that girls have continued on their first cycle, i.e. adopting smoking, whilst boys have entered the second cycle, namely adopting non-smoking. The stage has now been reached in Britain where very few people take up smoking after the age of 18-years[8]. It has become a children's habit. It must also not be forgotten that the children in the less affluent families are more likely than those from more affluent homes to have smoking parents. Children have long been known to be more likely to become smokers if their parents smoke[9] and are also subjected to exposure to environmental tobacco smoke in the home. Thus, the 'family circle' mentioned earlier is focused on the less affluent groups. The *Health of the Nation* document[10] sets out the targets for reducing lung cancer and also specifically for reducing the prevalence of smoking among 11 to 15-year-olds. The overall target of reducing smoking prevalence among 11 to 15-year-olds from 8%, as it was in 1988, to 6% in 1994 has not been reached[11]. If Rogers and Shoemaker's theory is to be applied, the target of reducing regular smoking is probably not appropriate to this age group. Reduction of incidence rather than reduction of prevalence would be the best measure of progress. Much

Table 1   Smoking behaviour in 11 to 15-year-old school children by sex: England, 1982 to 1992

Smoking behaviour	1982	1984	1986	1988	1990	1992
Boys	%	%	%	%	%	%
Regular smoker	11	13	7	7	9	9
Occasional smoker	7	9	5	5	6	6
Used to smoke	11	11	10	8	7	6
Tried smoking	26	24	23	23	22	22
Never smoked	45	44	55	58	56	57
Base (=100%)	1460	1928	1676	1489	1643	1662
Girls	%	%	%	%	%	%
Regular smoker	11	13	12	9	11	10
Occasional smoker	9	9	5	5	6	7
Used to smoke	10	10	10	9	7	7
Tried smoking	22	22	19	19	18	19
Never smoked	49	46	53	59	58	57
Base (=100%)	1514	1689	1508	1529	1478	1626
Total	%	%	%	%	%	%
Regular smoker	11	13	10	8	10	10
Occasional smoker	8	9	5	5	6	7
Used to smoke	10	10	10	8	7	7
Tried smoking	24	23	21	21	20	20
Never smoked	47	45	54	58	57	57
Base (=100%)	2979	3658	3189	3018	3121	3295

From: Thomas M, Holroyd S, Goddard E. *Smoking among Secondary School Children in 1992*. An enquiry carried out by the Social Survey Division of OPCS on behalf of the Department of Health, the Welsh Office and the Scottish Office Home and Health Department. London: HMSO, 1993, (p 14, table 3.3).

better would be to have set out to delay onset of the behaviour and this has, in fact, been achieved even in 15-year-olds, although, as might be expected if the theory holds, the delay and reduction has been greater in boys than in girls. Table 1 shows changes in smoking prevalence in the 11 to 15-year-old age group since 1982, when regular national surveys of smoking in this age group began[11].

The situation is quite different in countries where social norms and status for women and girls are less emancipated than in Britain. Relatively few women and girls have yet taken up the habit and the communication of innovations has still reached only the innovators and some early adopters (Table 2), whilst the curve for men and boys is at a later stage of development[12,13]. However, the tobacco industry would have it otherwise and is aggressively marketing tobacco in order to move its adoption to the next phases. In these countries, there is a real opportunity to halt the diffusion process before it spreads to the other adopters. In this way, health activists could benefit from knowing about the experience in industrialised countries and could take action to prevent the process before it progresses further, thus reducing to a minimum the

Table 2 Data on smoking prevalence of 15-year-olds, drawn from six recent national studies and *The WHO Cross National Study of Children's Health Behaviour*, 1986

		Smoke daily	Smoke weekly	Smoke once per week or more	Smoke less than weekly	Do not smoke (have tried)	Have never smoked	Sample No.
All countries	M	14.4	4.4	22.3	6.4	39.9	34.2	>5754
	F	14.4	5.6	28.0	8.0	36.3	36.3	>5934
Australia	M	—	—	25.0	—	—	—	—
	F	—	—	28.0	—	—	—	—
Austria	M	11.8	6.5	—	10.3	43.3	28.2	476
	F	13.1	7.1	—	11.8	39.1	28.9	381
Belgium	M	16.6	5.0	—	5.1	32.7	40.6	603
	F	13.5	6.2	—	5.6	29.4	45.3	502
Canada*	M	17.4	—	—	—	—	—	—
	F	17.8	—	—	—	—	—	—
Finland	M	29.1	6.3	—	6.3	39.9	18.4	539
	F	20.1	7.4	—	10.1	36.8	25.6	543
Hungary	M	20.4	5.9	—	8.2	39.9	25.4	562
	F	14.1	6.8	—	8.2	42.2	28.7	704
Israel	M	5.7	3.5	—	3.5	30.9	56.4	402
	F	4.1	3.4	—	6.3	21.3	64.9	559
New Zealand	M	10.0	—	—	—	—	—	—
	F	20.0	—	—	—	—	—	—
Norway	M	16.2	4.1	—	9.1	43.2	27.4	627
	F	17.6	6.3	—	14.4	35.6	26.1	568
Scotland	M	14.7	2.6	—	3.6	39.8	39.2	771
	F	15.6	4.5	—	6.7	40.0	33.3	711
Sweden	M	8.7	5.7	—	7.6	47.0	31.1	541
	F	10.9	5.6	—	7.1	37.6	38.8	521
Switzerland	M	9.5	3.6	—	10.2	35.8	40.9	279
	F	10.5	4.4	—	11.3	29.3	44.4	341
USA [†]	M	—	—	24.0	—	—	—	—
	F	—	—	29.0	—	—	—	—
Wales	M	13.1	2.4	—	4.4	41.9	38.2	954
	F	15.1	5.2	—	4.4	41.2	34.1	1104
Wales & Scotland	M	—	—	18.0	—	—	—	—
	F	—	—	27.0	—	—	—	—

Figures in percentages; [†] 15- and 16-year-olds; *15- to 19-year-olds. The data have been collected from a variety of studies with differing methodologies. The WHO cross-national survey statistics are courtesy of Nutbeam, D. *Planning for a Smoke-Free Generation. Smoke-Free Europe*:p. 6[78]. The table is reproduced from: Charlton A, Moyer C, Melia P. *A Manual on Tobacco and Young People for the Industrialised World*. Geneva: UICC, 1990; p. 3[78].

epidemic of smoking-related diseases which is bound to follow as it has done in the industrialised world.

Smoking and the unborn child

Adult smoking affects children even before they are born and perhaps even before they are conceived[14]. It is now nearly 30 years since the first evidence of low birth weight associated with smoking in pregnancy was published[15] and, during that period, a tremendous body of research evidence has been amassed showing effects of maternal and paternal smoking on the unborn child. It is impossible in a short paper to cover the topic in detail. Many reviews of the effect of smoking on the fetus are available and the reader is referred to some of these[8,16,17]. It is, however, essential to provide a brief overview here of such an important set of effects of smoking on children's health.

Low birth weight is the term generally used in the context of smoking to mean small for gestational age. Babies who are small for gestational age are at greater risk of health problems in the neonatal and perinatal period and there is even some evidence to suggest that the effects of this disadvantage might be carried forward into childhood. Early studies rarely included any factors other than smoking in their analyses, and there was a time when the findings were questioned on the grounds that socio-economic status or other confounding factors could be operating. However, studies including socio-economic status, maternal age, weight, height and weight gain in pregnancy, sex and ethnicity of the baby have carried out multivariate analyses and have found that smoking has the strongest effect on birth weight[18,19].

Babies born to smoking mothers are, on average, 200 g lighter than those born to non-smoking mothers[20]. The effect is dose-related. Mothers who smoked 10–20 cigarettes per day during pregnancy have had lower birth weight babies than those who smoke less[21]. Recent techniques to assess the level of cotinine, a metabolite of nicotine in the maternal blood, have enabled this dose-response effect to be measured accurately and physiologically. One such study has shown that women with the highest levels of serum cotinine had babies whose birth weight was 441 g less than those with the lowest levels[22], this study also suggested a reduction of 12 g birth weight for every cigarette smoked per day.

The most marked effect on birth weight appears to be caused by maternal smoking during the second and third trimesters of pregnancy[23], which enables the mother to have a little leeway in stopping smoking when she knows she is pregnant. Unfortunately, pregnant women are a surprisingly difficult group with which to intervene. In spite of having so much reason to stop smoking, only a quarter succeed in stopping smoking at some time during pregnancy and about two-thirds of those who are successful take up smoking again after the birth[24]. Paternal smoking is also associated with babies being small for gestational age[25].

Spontaneous abortion of the fetus is more frequent in smoking than in non-smoking mothers[26], as is perinatal mortality[27].

It is, of course, difficult to separate the effects of pre- and post-natal exposure to smoke in many cases, because the mothers who smoke in pregnancy are likely also to smoke in the home as their infant is growing up. Perhaps the most important of these dual effects is that of the sudden infant death syndrome (SIDS). A valuable analysis[28] of the findings of ten recent major studies on this topic found that all except one showed an association between maternal smoking during pregnancy and increased incidence of SIDS. Most of the studies took other social factors into account, such as maternal age, parity, housing conditions, marital status, education and unemployment and found that smoking was still a significant factor. Sleeping position was not taken into account in these studies.

Other possible serious health risks in the life of a child, who was exposed to smoke during his or her fetal development, include cancers. A number of studies on maternal smoking during pregnancy and risk of childhood cancer have been carried out over the past 25 years, but their outcomes are still inconclusive. Because childhood cancers are relatively infrequent, the small numbers have caused problems, in general, with analysis and interpretation of results.

Out of three cohort studies, only one has found a significant link between maternal smoking during pregnancy and increased risk of childhood cancer. The earliest of these studies, in 1971, found little evidence of increased risk[29], and the most recently reported in 1992[30], found no increase in the overall cancer risk in children whose mothers smoked during pregnancy (relative risk 0.99; 95% CI 0.78–1.27). This study was a survey of 497,051 children born in Sweden between 1982 and 1987. There were 198 solid tumours and 129 lymphatic/haematopoietic cancers. Risks for solid tumours were also not increased (relative risk 0.96; 95% CI 0.70–1.32) but cancers of the lymphatic/haematopoietic system showed a relative risk of 1.04; 95% CI 0.71–1.52. The risk did not increase with the number of cigarettes smoked each day by the mother. No significant site specific increase in risk was found for solid tumours or lymphatic/haematopoietic cancers. The third cohort study[31] published in 1990 examined data from the British Birth Cohort (BCS70) where 33 children out of 16,193 born in one week in April 1970 developed cancers (2.04 per 1000 births). Here, logistic regression involving the whole cohort found an independent statistical association between childhood cancer and maternal smoking during pregnancy (OR 2.5).

Case control studies have also yielded equivocal results. In 1986, another Swedish study[32] of 305 children with cancer and a control group of 340 children with diabetes mellitus found a 50% increase in overall cancer risk for the children exposed to 10 or more cigarettes per day during pregnancy. They also found an increase for single sites, including a doubling of risk for Wilms' tumour, Hodgkin's lymphoma and acute lymphoblastic leukaemia. However, the reaction to this publication was swift, with a British Inter-Regional Epidemiological Study of Childhood

Cancers (IRESCC) study[33] of 555 cases, each with two matched controls, showing no increased risk of cancers in children of mothers who smoked during pregnancy. The US Children's Cancer Study Group (CCSG) also responded with a study showing that they found no significant increase[34].

In 1991, another case control study[35], in Denver, Colorado involved children aged 0–14 years, born from 1976–1983. There were 223 cases and 196 controls. However, the diagnostic subgroups were very small and the authors advised caution in interpreting the findings. Mother's smoking in the first trimester, when adjusted for father's education, was found to be associated with increased risk of cancers in general (OR 1.3, 95% CI 0.7–2.1), acute lymphocytic leukaemia (OR 1.9, 95% CI 0.9–4.1) and lymphomas (OR 2.3, 95% CI 0.8–7.1). When father's smoking during his partner's pregnancy was considered, and adjusted for his educational status, some increased risk was found for the same three cancer groups. An increased risk of brain cancer was also identified (OR 1.4; 95% CI 0.7–3.5), which is interesting in view of a later study which also found an increased risk related to paternal smoking[36].

All these studies advise caution in interpretation due to small numbers and numerous confounding factors and methodological limitations and variations. The situation with regard to maternal and passive smoking and childhood cancer is an important one which merits further investigation.

Returning to the premise of a 'family circle' in the children of smokers, the effects of exposure to smoke during fetal development can be summed up in two ways: the dramatic acute effects causing death of the child and the continuing chronic effects which can affect the child's life in many ways in the future. To end this section, it is appropriate to review these less spectacular effects which can undermine a child's social and academic development. They fall into three groups as follows: minor ailments; effects on growth; effects on academic achievement. With regard to the first of these, *in utero* exposure to smoke has been found to be strongly related to an increased incidence of respiratory illnesses in children[37], over and above the effects of exposure to passive smoking in the home. Growth is also less in children of smoking mothers, several studies having found that children of smokers are shorter and lighter in weight at the ages of 5-[38] and 7-years[39], which is consistent with the development of low birth weight children in general. Small stature is likely to affect children's self-esteem and impede their social development. Finally, there is evidence that babies born to smokers have a smaller head circumference[40], suggesting that exposure to smoke during fetal development might restrict brain growth. Further evidence for this is found in young adults in a national cohort study where lower academic achievement was linked to mother's smoking during pregnancy even when other factors such as social class were taken into account[41]. So the child of a smoker starts life with several disadvantages, which can then be compounded if family smoking continues during his or her infancy and childhood.

Family smoking and the health risks to children

Children who are brought up in homes where the parents smoke have little or no choice with regard to their own exposure to smoke. Infants at home with their mother are in an especially vulnerable position. Early studies focused on infants and the frequency of respiratory disease, sometimes associated with admissions to hospital. A review of studies with large data sets carried out since the late 1970s was published in 1992[42]. Whilst the sampling and methodology of the studies varied considerably, the outcomes were generally consistent in finding an increased risk of respiratory problems in children of smoking parents. However, an analysis of data from the British Birth Cohort Study (BCS70) in this same publication shed more light on the pre- and post-natal nature of the various symptoms[42]. In mothers who had smoked in pregnancy, the history of wheezing and bronchitis in the children measured at either 5- or 10-years was significantly increased, as was snoring and habitual mouth-breathing at the age of 5-years. Children of multiparae had a more frequent history of pneumonia at the age of 5-years, and of cough and shortness of breath at the age of 10-years. The authors of this study also considered mothers who did not smoke in pregnancy, but smoked post-natally. In this case, the only respiratory symptoms which were significantly more frequent in their children compared with those of non-smokers were habitual snoring and mouth-breathing at 5-years, sore throats at 5-years and coughs at 10-years which were of borderline significance. When the same respiratory symptoms were studied in the children of smoking mothers who smoked throughout pregnancy, those who did not and non-smokers, only snoring and mouth-breathing was significantly higher in those who did not smoke in pregnancy. The authors concluded that maternal smoking in pregnancy was linked to an increase in the child's risk of wheezing, bronchitis and pneumonia and post-natal exposure to smoke to increased risk of habitual snoring and mouth-breathing and perhaps of chronic coughs. They also concluded that exposure to passive smoking post-natally has a more marked effect on problems of the upper respiratory tract than on lower respiratory problems.

This study has been considered more fully than others here, because it attempts to untangle the pre- and post-natal effects. There is, however, a considerable body of evidence which reinforces these findings and covers a considerable number of other health risks in children who are exposed to passive smoking at home. The effect of exposure to environmental tobacco smoke in the home is particularly problematic for children with asthma, by increasing the frequency and severity of symptoms[43], thus compounding effects of *in utero* exposure. The incidence of middle ear effusion[44] and sore throats[45], also greatly increased in children who are exposed to smoke in the home.

Passive smoking is, therefore, a cog in the 'family circle'. The children who are exposed to it are likely to suffer from more minor ailments than those who have smoke-free homes. Minor ailments cause absence from school, or underperformance. A study of 2,800 schoolchildren aged 12–13-years[46] found that the risk of being absent from school on a randomly selected day was not only related to the children's own smoking behaviour, but the risk was increased by equal amounts if the mother also smoked. Motivation falls if the continuity of learning is frequently broken. It becomes difficult to keep up with the rest of the class, self-esteem or self-perception falls in this domain. It is well-known that those children who underachieve, who are 'fed up' with school and who place little value on academic progress are the most likely to take up smoking. A recent study showed that low self-perception in the scholastic achievement domain in boys and girls, measured by Harter's Self-Perception Profile for Children[47], was most significantly related to being a smoker[48]. Another link is then forged in the chain from adult to child to adult. Not only has the children's health been harmed, they are now on their way to damaging their own health even further.

In fact, the same three disadvantages of minor ailments, growth[49,50], and probably academic development, are compounded by exposure to environmental tobacco smoke during childhood. These children are also at the greatest risk of becoming smokers themselves. The question of lung cancer in adults who were exposed to environmental tobacco smoke in their homes during childhood is a difficult one, due to the very long latent period between exposure and appearance of lesions and symptoms. Several studies have attempted to tease out the answer. The earliest reported case-control study on this topic involving 1338 lung cancer patients and 1393 comparison subjects found that, when variables indicative of active smoking were controlled for in a logistic regression analysis, exposure to maternal smoke was associated with an increased risk of lung cancer in smokers. The relative risk for both sexes was 1.36 ($p<0.02$) and for males was 1.5 ($p<0.01$). No increased risk was found for females or for subjects whose father smoked. The authors emphasised the preliminary nature of these findings and the possibility of confounding factors which were not controlled for[51]. Two years later a study of 518 patients from a hospital-based tumour registry found that the overall risk of cancers rose by 60% for those exposed in childhood only, by 50%

for those exposed in adulthood only, but more than doubled (OR 2.7) for those exposed in both childhood and adulthood[52]. Trends were similar for smokers (who had smoked at least one cigarette for a period of at least six months) and non-smokers.

A more recent study of lung cancer patients[53], showed that exposure to 25 or more 'smoker years', e.g. living with two smokers for 12.5 years during childhood and adolescence appeared to double the risk of lung cancer in those patients who have never smoked.

More investigation on the possibly increased risk of lung cancer in people exposed to environmental tobacco smoke as children is needed.

The health risks of a child's own smoking

There is always a tendency to consider only the serious long-term risks to health which are posed by personal smoking. However, for children, the immediate or short-term risks are not only very relevant in practical terms, they are also much more meaningful as a possible deterrent. Such risks as lung cancer and heart diseases which usually affect older people seem too far ahead to be of any relevance to a young smoker. Immediate discomfort can far outweigh the extension of life even by a few years. After all, when one is really old, what is the benefit of living to be even older, they think. It cannot be any fun.

Coughs and respiratory problems do start to occur immediately. A survey of 16,000 young people in the UK in the 1980s found that, even from the age of 10-years, young smokers of one cigarette per week or more were more likely than non-smokers to report frequent coughs[54]. Whilst the incidence of frequent coughs fell steadily overall as the children became older, the increased risk among smokers remained high (Fig. 3). As long ago as the 1970s, Bewley *et al.*[55] showed that the risk of respiratory symptoms in young smokers in the 10- to 12-year-old age group was double that of non-smokers. In both these studies, young smokers were defined as smoking at least one cigarette per week. Numerous other studies have shown increased risk of cough, wheeze, shortness of breath and increase of sputum[8]. The increase in risk appears to be the same whether low or middle tar cigarettes are smoked[56].

Lung function can also be affected in young smokers[57–59]. A study of 669 young people, aged 5- to 19-years at the start, who were followed up annually for changes in FEV in one second (FEV_1) and FEF_{25-75} (forced expiratory flow during the middle half of vital capacity), found significant decreases in both measures associated with smoking. When previous FEV_1 and FEF_{25-75}, age, sex, height and mother's smoking were controlled for, personal smoking was associated with significant

Percent

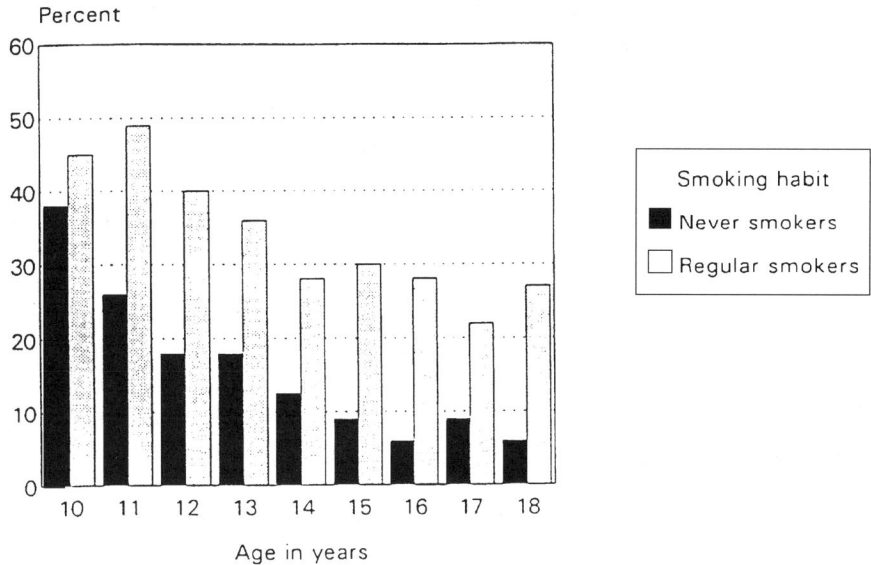

Fig. 3 Self-reported frequent coughs in 10- to 18-year-olds in never-smokers and in regular smokers of one or more cigarettes per week. (Reference: Charlton A. The Brigantia Smoking Survey: a general review. *Public Education about Cancer* 1984; 77: 92–102)

decreases in FEV_1 ($p<0.001$) and FEF_{25-75} ($p=0.033$). On this basis, the authors estimated that starting to smoke at the age of 15 would reduce FEV_1 to 92% and FEF_{25-75} to 90% of the expected by the age of 20. Very interestingly, one study has found that children who take up smoking appear to have higher levels of lung function at that stage, but 5 years of smoking reduces it to the same level as that of non-smokers[59]. However, there is evidence, in a study of 10 young doctors who smoked, that after 3 weeks of abstinence from smoking, peak expiratory flow (PEF) was significantly increased[60]. Similar findings occurred among 195 boys during 8 weeks at a detention centre where they were not allowed to smoke[61], all except the heaviest smokers having near normal PEF at the end of the 8 weeks. It does, therefore, appear that the reduction in PEF can be reversed by quitting smoking.

Fitness levels are also immediately affected due to the replacement of oxygen by carbon monoxide in the haemoglobin. Addiction is also an important element in the immediate effects of smoking. Young people tend either to dismiss it on the grounds that it takes a long time to develop, will not happen to them and that they can easily give up smoking whenever they want to, or they actually **like** the idea of being addicted. Research has shown that the addiction process quickly takes hold. Much evidence of addiction in young people is provided by the research carried out by McNeill, in two valuable studies: one showed that young smokers, deprived of cigarettes, experience withdrawal symptoms associated with addiction to nicotine[62] and the second showing that inhalation of smoke occurs early in a smoker's experience, thus emphasising the importance of the first few cigarettes[63]. These findings confirm that addiction can be established quickly and at an early age. A national survey in the UK found that 65% of 16- to 19-year-old smokers had made at least one attempt to stop smoking[64] and half of these young people had made more than one attempt and failed. Another study found that three-quarters of smokers aged 16- to 19-years had tried to stop, 4% of them had first tried, unsuccessfully, at the age of 12 years[65].

Blood pressure presents an interesting picture with regard to young smokers. There is a considerable body of research evidence which indicates that adult smokers, including young smokers, have lower mean blood pressure and pulse rate than non-smokers[66–72], but smoking a cigarette raises the heart rate within 1 min, with perhaps as much as a 30% increase in 10 min[73]. Blood pressure also increases sharply by 7–10% due to peripheral vasoconstriction and changes in the regional blood flow. Recent research raises the question as to whether or not low blood pressure might precede the uptake of smoking in children, but this issue requires further investigation and interpretation[74].

There are many other immediate or short-term effects of active smoking on children including increased risk of leukoplakia[75], greater susceptibility to infection due to decreased immunity[76], damage to the cilia lining the trachea, shaky hands and increased pulse rate, all of which to a greater or lesser extent are experienced by the child. However, the basis for life-threatening diseases later in life is already being laid down in young smokers. There is evidence that smoking started before the age of 15-years greatly increases the risk of lung cancer in later life[77,78]. The forerunners of cardio-vascular diseases can already be observed in increased likelihood of the blood to clot, changes in blood lipids, and evidence of atherosclerosis[8].

The health effects as well as the family norms have conspired to make the 'at risk' children more likely to be smokers. They leave school as early as possible, having failed to achieve their maximum potential, and they are likely to have early pregnancies. There is evidence that younger women with a lower educational attainment, working in unskilled jobs are most likely to smoke during pregnancy, as are their male partners. Thus the cycle is continued to the next generation of children. The 'family circle' is complete.

Children of smoking mothers, especially those who smoke during pregnancy, are more likely than children of non-smokers to have health problems, which can cause them to miss time from school and fall behind with their work. Children who feel they are not achieving academically are at increased risk of taking up smoking. They are also more likely to take up smoking due to the norms of their family.

Prevention issues

How can this family circle be broken? Since the health risks of smoking were first published 40 years ago, this problem has been considered. The early attempts were largely academic in approach and often school-based. They were, not unexpectedly, largely unsuccessful on the basis that it is the least academically inclined young people who are most likely to take up smoking and to be the late majority or even the laggards in the communication of innovations process to adopt non-smoking. School-based education has not been entirely unsuccessful and sets of guidelines based on research outcomes have been developed[79,80]. Social skills and short-term, rather than long-term, health risks form the best content; peer-teaching, parental involvement for younger children and sufficient time allocation (10 sessions in the critical 2-year period following the peak initiation age is suggested) have all been shown to increase effectiveness. However, the best which can be achieved in this way appears to be a delay in onset rather than a decrease in prevalence in regular smokers. This reservation has serious implications for the target set in *The Health of the Nation,* as was mentioned earlier in this paper. Perhaps the most serious shortfall in school-based education is that it fails to reach the 'drop outs' as the early school-leavers are called in the US[81]. As has been discussed, these young people are most at risk and are most likely to form 'family circles' of the type discussed in this paper. They must be reached in other less academic ways. Many are anti-establishment. Having failed to attain the targets which are usually set by the establishment, they reject these norms and rebel against them. Rebelliousness is a major factor in the uptake of smoking by young people[82]. These young people are, therefore, unlikely to attend youth clubs because these are also establishment-based. They are unlikely to join Smokebuster clubs or similar out-of-school organised activities. The points at which the circle can be broken need more practical action.

If the 'family circle' of smoking is to be broken, the time for information, education and advice is past. What is now needed is positive action to help. In summary, some suggested actions for consideration which arise out of this review of children's health and smoking are tentatively presented as follows:

1. Prophylactic medical help for the 'at risk' infants, children and young people in the form of dietary supplements such as vitamins C and D, and provision of medication and immunization for children identified as being 'at risk' as a result of screening at post-natal clinics, and by midwives, community nurses and school nurses. Children's health should not be penalized because their parents smoke. Help now is

likely to prevent them from taking up smoking later and could prevent the health problems from arising.

2. Pre-pregnancy provision of nicotine replacement therapy at preparation for parenthood classes, provided that such a therapy can be developed and recommended for safe use with the appropriate age group.

3. Family approaches through ante- and post-natal clinics, day care centres, schools and other appropriate channels to raise self-esteem, to strengthen coping, to identify **why** smoking outweighs family and personal health, and to develop shared methods of overcoming these problems or needs. Ownership of the programmes by the families themselves is essential. Programmes should not be imposed from outside by non-smoking health educators who think they know how the families feel. If social help is needed, it must be provided.

4. Government action is also needed to ban cigarette advertising and to create a smoke-free norm.

Action, not leaflets, is needed to break the 'family circle' of smoking.

As a recent paper emphasises, the lifestyle of smokers may differ widely from that of non-smokers, smoking is only one part of this lifestyle and health and development problems in the children may be influenced by this complex interaction[83]. Women who smoke need help in coping with the stresses of their lives.

Acknowledgement

The author wishes to thank the Cancer Research Campaign for funding her research.

References

1   Rogers EM, Shoemaker FF. *Communications of Innovations*. New York: Free Press, 1971

2   US Department of Health and Human Services. *The Health Consequences of Smoking. A Report by the Surgeon General*. US Department of Health and Human Services, Public Health Service, Office on Smoking and Health, Rockville, Maryland, USA, 1982

3   Charlton A, Moyer C, Mackay J, Lam TH, Niu S. *Smoking and Youth in China, 1992*. Geneva: International Union Against Cancer, 1993

4   Royal College of Physicians. *Smoking and Health*. A report on smoking in relation to lung cancer and other diseases. London: Pitman Medical, 1962

5   Thomas M, Goddard E, Hickman M, Hunter P. *General Household Survey 1992*. Series GHS No 23. London: HMSO, 1994

6   Royal College of Physicians. *Smoking or Health*. London: Pitman Medical, 1977

7   Bynner JM. *The Young Smoker*. London: HMSO, 1969

8   Royal College of Physicians. *Smoking and the Young.* London: The Royal College of Physicians, 1992

9   Bewley BP, Bland JM, Harris R. Factors associated with the starting of cigarette smoking by primary school children. *Br J Prev Soc Med* 1974; **28**: 37–44

10 Secretary of State for Health of Her Majesty's Government. *The Health of the Nation.* London: HMSO, 1992

11 Thomas M, Holroyd S, Goddard E. *Smoking among Secondary School Children in 1992.* London: HMSO, 1993

12 Peto R, Lopez AD, Boreham J, Thun M, Heath C. *Mortality from Smoking in Developed Countries 1950–2000.* Oxford: Oxford University Press, 1994

13 Charlton A, Moyer C. *et al.* (Eds.) *Children and Tobacco: the wider view.* Geneva: International Union Against Cancer, 1991

14 Davis DL. Paternal smoking and fetal health. *Lancet* 1991; **337**: 123

15 Simpson WJ. A preliminary report of cigarette smoking and the incidence of prematurity. *Am J Obstet Gynecol* 1957; **73**: 808–15

16 Poswillo D, Alberman E. (Eds). *Effects of Smoking on the Fetus, Neonate and Child.* Oxford: Oxford University Press, 1992

17 Charlton A. Children and passive smoking: a review. *J Fam Pract* 1994; **38**: 267–77

18 Brooke OG, Anderson HR, Bland JM, Peacock JL, Stewart C. Effect on birth weight of smoking, alcohol, caffeine, socio-economic factors and psychosocial stress. *BMJ* 1989; **298**: 795–801

19 Abell TD, Baker LC, Ramsey CN. The effects of maternal smoking on infant birth weight. *Fam Med* 1991; **23**: 103–7

20 Stein Z, Klein J. Smoking, alcohol and reproduction. *Am J Public Health* 1983; **73**: 1154–6

21 Meyer M, Jonas B, Tonascia J. Perinatal events associated with maternal smoking. *Am J Epidemiol* 1976; **103**: 464–76

22 Haddow JE, Knight GJ, Palomaki GE, Kloza BM, Wald NJ. Cigarette consumption and serum cotinine in relation to birth weight. *Br J Obstet Gynaecol* 1987; **94**: 678–81

23 MacArthur C, Knox EG. Smoking in pregnancy: effects of stopping at different stages. *Br J Obstet Gynaecol* 1988; **95**: 551–5

24 Gillies PA, Madeley RJ, Power FL. Smoking cessation in pregnancy – a controlled trial of the impact of new technology and friendly encouragement. In: Aoki M, Hisamichi S, Tominaga S. (Eds) *Smoking and Health 1987.* Amsterdam: Elsevier, 1988

25 Rubin DH, Krasilnikoff PA, Leventhal JM, Weile W, Berget A. Effect of passive smoking on birth weight. *Lancet* 1986; **ii**: 415–17

26 Himmelberger D, Brown B, Cohen E. Cigarette smoking during pregnancy and the occurrence of spontaneous abortion and congenital abnormality. *Am J Epidemiol* 1978; **108**: 470–9

27 Butler NR, Goldstein H, Ross EM. Cigarette smoking in pregnancy: its influence on birth weight and perinatal mortality. *BMJ* 1972; **2**: 127–30

28 Nicholl J, O'Cathain A. Antenatal smoking, postnatal passive smoking and the Sudden Infant Death Syndrome. In: Poswillo D, Alberman E. (Eds) *Effects of Smoking on the Fetus, Neonate and Child.* Oxford: Oxford University Press, 1992

29 Neutel CI, Buck C. Effect of smoking during pregnancy on the risk of cancer in children. *J Natl Cancer Inst* 1971; **47**: 59–63

30 Pershagen G, Ericson A, Otterblad-Olausson P. Maternal smoking in pregnancy: does it increase the risk of childhood cancer? *Int J Epidemiol* 1992; **21**: 1–5

31 Golding J, Paterson M, Kinlen LJ. Factors associated with child cancer in a national cohort study. *Br J Cancer* 1990; **62**: 304–8

32 Stjernfeldt M, Berglund K, Lindsten J, Ludvigson J. Maternal smoking during pregnancy and risk of childhood cancer. *Lancet* 1986; **i**: 1350–52

33 McKinney PA, Stiller CA. Maternal smoking during pregnancy and the risk of childhood cancer. *Lancet* 1986; **ii**: 519

34 Buckley JD, Hobbie WL, Ruccione K *et al.* Maternal smoking during pregnancy and the risk of childhood cancer. *Lancet* 1986; **ii**: 519–20

35 John EM, Savitz DA, Sandler DP. Prenatal exposure to parents' smoking and childhood cancer. *Am J Epidemiol* 1991; **133**: 123–32

36 McCredie M, Maisonneuve P, Boyle P. Antenatal risk factors for malignant brain tumours in New South Wales children. *Int J Cancer* 1994; **56**: 6–10

37 Taylor B, Wadsworth J. Maternal smoking during pregnancy and lower respiratory tract illness in early life. *Arch Dis Child* 1987; **66**: 786–91

38 Elwood PC, Sweetnam PM, Gray OP, Davies DP, Wood PD. Growth of children from 0–5 years: with special reference to mothers' smoking in pregnancy. *Ann Hum Biol* 1987; **14**: 92–111

39 Goldstein H. Factors influencing the height of seven-year-old children. *Hum Biol* 1971; **43**: 92–111

40 D'Souza SW, Black P, Richards B. Smoking in pregnancy: association with skinfold thickness, maternal weight gain and foetal size at birth. *BMJ* 1981; **282**: 1661–3

41 Fogelman KR, Manor O. Smoking in pregnancy and development into early adulthood. *BMJ* 1988; **297**: 1233–6

42 Evans J-A, Golding J. Parental smoking and respiratory problems in childhood. In: Poswillo D, Alberman E. (Eds) *Effects of Smoking on the Fetus, Neonate and Child*. Oxford: Oxford University Press, 1992

43 Weitzman M, Gortmacker SL, Walker DK, Sobol A. Maternal smoking and childhood asthma. *Pediatrics* 1990; **35**: 505–11

44 Kraemer MJ, Marshall SG, Richardson MA. Etiologic factors in the development of chronic middle ear effusions. *Clin Rev Allergy* 1984; **2**: 319–28

45 Willatt DJ. Children's sore throats related to parental smoking. *Clin Otolaryngol* 1986; **11**: 317–21

46 Charlton A, Blair V. Absence from school related to children's and parental smoking habits. *BMJ* 1989; **298**: 90–2

47 Harter S. *Manual for the Self-Perception Profile for Children*. Denver, Colorado: University of Denver, 1985

48 Minagawa K, While D, Charlton A. Smoking and self-perception in secondary school students. *Tobacco Control* 1993; **2**: 215–21

49 Berkey SC, Ware JH, Speizer FE, Ferris BG. Passive smoking and height growth of preadolescent children. *Int J Epidemiol* 1984; **13**: 454–8

50 Rona RJ, Chinn S, Florey CD. Exposure to cigarette smoking and children's growth. *Int J Epidemiol* 1985; **14**: 402–9

51 Correa P, Pickle LW, Fontham E, Lin Y, Haenszel W. Passive smoking and lung cancer. *Lancet* 1983; **2**: 595–7

52 Sandler DP, Wilcox AJ, Everson RB. Cumulative effects of lifetime passive smoking on cancer risk. *Lancet* 1985; **i**: 312–15

53 Janerich DT, Thompson WD, Varela LR *et al*. Lung cancer and exposure to tobacco smoke in the household. *N Engl J Med* 1990; **323**: 632–6

54 Charlton A. Children's coughs related to parental smoking. *BMJ* 1984; **288**: 1647–9

55 Bewley BR, Halil T, Snaith AH. Smoking by primary school children: prevalence and associated respiratory symptoms. *Br J Prev Soc Med* 1973; **27**: 150–3

56 Rimpela AH, Rimpela MK. Increased risk of respiratory symptoms in young smokers of low tar cigarettes. *BMJ* 1985; **290**: 1461–3

57 Tager IB, Munoz A, Rosner B, Weiss St, Carey V, Speizer FE. Effect of cigarette smoking on the pulmonary function of children and adolescents. *Am Rev Resp Dis* 1985; **131**: 752–9

58 Walter S, Nancy NR, Collier CR. Changes in forced expiratory spirogram in young male smokers. *Am Rev Respir Dis* 1979; **119**: 117–24.

59 Tashkin DP, Clark VA, Coulson AH *et al*. Comparison of lung function in young nonsmokers and smokers before and after initiation of the smoking habit. A prospective study. *Am Rev Respir Dis* 1983; **128**: 12–16

60 Krumholz RA, Chevalier RB, Ross JC. Changes in cardiopulmonary functions related to abstinence from smoking: studies in young cigarette smokers and rest and exercise at 3 and 6 weeks after abstinence. *Ann Intern Med* 1965; **6**: 197–207

61 Backhouse CI. Peak flow in youths with varying cigarette habits. *BMJ* 1975; **1**: 360–2

62 McNeill AD, West RJ, Jarvis MJ, Jackson P, Russell MAH. Cigarette withdrawal symptoms in adolescent smokers. *Psychopharmacology* 1986; **90**: 533–6

63 McNeill AD. The development of dependence on smoking in children. *Br J Addict* 1991; **86**: 589–92

64 Marsh A, Matheson J. *Smoking Attitudes and Behaviour*. London: HMSO, 1983

65 Charlton A. Smoking cessation in schools and colleges. *J Smoking Rel Disorders* 1995; **5**: 289–94

66 Berglund G, Wilhelmsen L. Factors related to blood pressure in a general population sample of Swedish men. *Acta Med Scand* 1975; **198**: 291–8

67 Erikssen J, Enger SC. The effect of smoking on selected coronary heart disease risk factors in middle-aged men. *Acta Med Scand* 1978; **203**: 27–30

68 Stamler J, Rhomberg P, Schoenberger JA *et al*. Multivariate analysis of the relationship of seven variables to blood pressure. Findings of the Chicago Heart Association Detection Project in Industry 1967–1972. *J Chron Dis* 1975; **28**: 527–48

69 Kesteloot H, Van Houte O. An epidemiologic survey of arterial blood pressure in a large male population group. *Am J Epidemiol* 1974; **99**: 14–29

70 Gyntelberg F, Meyer J. Relationship between blood pressure, physical fitness, smoking and alcohol consumption in Copenhagen males aged 40–59. *Acta Med Scand* 1974; **195**: 375–80

71 Green MS, Jucha E, Luz Y. Blood pressure in smokers and nonsmokers: epidemiologic findings *Am Heart J* 1986; **111**: 932–40

72 Townsend J, Wilkes H, Haines A, Jarvis M. Adolescent smokers seen in general practice: health, lifestyle, physical measurements and response to antismoking advice. *BMJ* 1991; **303**: 947–50 (correction *BMJ* 1991; **303**: 1553)

73 Trap-Jensen J. Effects of smoking on the heart and peripheral circulation. *Am Heart J* 1988; **115**: 263–6

74 Charlton A, While D. Blood pressure and smoking: observations on a national cohort. *Arch Dis Childhood* 1995; In press

75 Von Wyk CW. An oral pathology profile of a group of juvenile delinquents. *J Forensic Odontostomatol* 1983; **1**: 3–10

76 Holt PG. Immune and inflammatory function in cigarette smokers. *Thorax* 1987; **42**: 241–9

77 Peto R. Influence of dose and duration of smoking on lung cancer rates. In: Zarridge DG, Peto R. (Eds) *Tobacco: a Major International Health Hazard*. Lyon, France: International Agency for Research on Cancer, 1986: 23–33

78 US Department of Health and Human Services. *The Health Consequences of Smoking: Cancer. A Report of the Surgeon General*. US Department of Health and Human Services, Public Health Service, Office on Smoking and Health, Rockville, MD, USA

79 Glynn T. Essential elements of school-based smoking prevention programmes. *J School Health* 1989; **59**: 181–8

80 Bruvold WH. A meta-analysis of adolescent smoking prevention programs. *Am J Public Health* 1993; **83**: 872–80

81 Charlton A, Moyer C, Melia P. *A Manual on Tobacco and Young People for the Industrialised World*. Geneva: UICC, 1990

82 Steward L, Livson N. Smoking and rebelliousness: a longitudinal study from childhood to maturity. *J Consult Lin Psychol* 1966; **30**: 225–9

83 Rantakallio P, Läärä E, Koiranen M. A 28 year follow up of mortality among women who smoked during pregnancy. *BMJ* 1995; **311**: 477–80

Tobacco control: overview

Donald Reid

Association for Public Health, London, UK

This chapter assesses the principal components of an effective tobacco control programme in relation to efficacy, reach (i.e. numbers of smokers influenced) and cost-effectiveness. National targets for the reduction of prevalence are most likely to be achieved through the use of high reach interventions such as fiscal policy and mass communications.

Restrictions on smoking at work may contribute to declines in consumption, but advice from health professionals, though effective, has limited impact owing to low reach. Measures aimed primarily at youth can delay, but not prevent, recruitment to smoking.

Media publicity not only reduces smoking, but also creates a climate of opinion in favour of effective measures such as fiscal policy. In the long run, health professionals can achieve more for their patients through the media than through personal advice.

The purpose of this chapter is to identify and appraise the principal components of an effective national tobacco control programme, based on experience in the UK and similar countries. The first step in the design of an effective programme is to set measurable targets, together with dates for their achievement. Prevalence is the most useful indicator for this purpose, with per caput consumption as a secondary measure[1]. For example, the UK Government's principal target is to reduce prevalence by one-third by the year 2000 (relative to a 1990 baseline)[2], across the UK as a whole. It is supported by targets for youth, pregnant women, and overall consumption. Since these cannot be set without reliable data, the UK Government conducts biennial prevalence surveys with samples of up to 20,000 adults and 3,000 teenagers, and provides annual data on consumption. It also measures implementation of the strategy and the state of public opinion[3].

Available interventions

In addition to surveys, the principal components of an effective strategy[4] include legislation[5] to ban tobacco advertising and sales to youth, provision of health education, use of fiscal policy (i.e. taxation) to increase cigarette prices, and restrictions on smoking in public places. Other measures include product modification through regulation of tar and nicotine content[5], and removal of subsidies to growers[5] (which has the same effect as fiscal policy and is therefore not discussed further). All of these actions are effective to varying degrees. However, since resources are always limited, it is important to identify the most effective options, based on defined criteria.

Criteria for appraisal

If national targets are to be met, large numbers of people must be influenced within a short period of time. For example, achievement of the UK year 2000 prevalence target requires an annual decline of 500,000 in a smoking population of 15 million, equivalent to 380,000 for England only[3]. Consequently, the criteria on which this appraisal is based include **reach** – the proportion of the target population likely to be reached by an intervention within a defined period, as well as **efficacy** – the extent of any effect on prevalence. As far as possible, evidence for efficacy is based on quit rates at one year follow up, validated biochemically. Where appropriate, **cost-effectiveness** from a health sector perspective has been included, using UK data which are not necessarily applicable elsewhere.

The combination of efficacy and reach provides a measure of overall **impact**[6]; the most effective interventions are those which achieve greatest impact for the lowest cost to the health sector. The interventions to be appraised (Table 1) are grouped into categories according to their principal purpose – prevention, cessation or general.

Prevention: interventions aimed primarily at youth

Despite the allocation of substantial resources to prevention, teenage prevalence has remained relatively unchanged in the UK and elsewhere during the last decade, despite concurrent declines in adult prevalence. In the UK, 1 in 4 teenagers become regular smokers by the age of 16, with the bulk of recruitment between ages 12–15[6]. Interventions to prevent teenage smoking include school health education, the use of the mass media and restrictions on sales to children[6].

School health education

Controlled trials, chiefly in the USA, have shown that the provision of information on smoking and health has no effect on teenage prevalence[7].

Table 1 Summary of principal interventions

Intervention	Efficacy: effects on prevalence and consumption	Cost–effectiveness in US$ (from a health sector perspective)	Reach (i.e. extent to which intervention can reach large number of smokers quickly)	Comments
A. Prevention: interventions aimed primarily at youth				
1. School health education	Can delay recruitment for several years, but not indefinitely	Minimal costs; effectiveness under real life conditions is uncertain	Limited: effective programmes are difficult to implement	Delay is useful, but overall impact is limited
2. Restrictions on smoking in schools	Uncertain	Minimal costs	Can be difficult to implement effectively	Desirable in order to set an example
3. Clubs for non-smoking teenagers ('Smoke Busters' Clubs)	Possible delaying effect, but evidence is weak	Poor in terms of direct effects on smoking	Can recruit large numbers in particular localities	Not recommended except for publicity generation
4. Cessation programmes for teenagers	Poor	Poor	Low	Not recommended
5. Mass campaigns	40% fall in prevalence in Vermont trial; no effect in Minnesota or England	Low: in range $233–1135 per delayed smoker (Vermont)	Very high	Unlikely to be as cost-effective as other options
6. Restrictions on sales to teenagers	Vigorous activity can reduce sales locally; possible delaying effect	Minimal cost to health sector	Low in UK to date	Can be a useful source of publicity
B. Interventions aimed at adults				
7. Smokers' advice clinics	10–25% quit rate	Low relative to other interventions	Very low	Only justified in special circumstances
8. Telephone 'Quit Lines'	19% quit rate at 6 months in Scotland with mass campaign	$150 per quitter in Scotland	High if well advertised and calls are free	Potentially high impact if part of mass campaign
9. Brief advice from a GP	Up to 5% quit rate	Highly cost-effective: in range $18–150 per year of life saved (YLS)	Relatively low in UK to date	Highly cost-effective but under used. More elaborate GP interventions are less cost effective
10. Nicotine replacement therapy (NRT)	Significantly enhances effectiveness of GP advice	Cost of GP advice to smoker to purchase patch in range $36–300 per YLS	Price may deter some smokers	Not as cost-effective as brief advice, but may be desirable with highly dependent smokers
11. Restrictions on smoking in the workplace	Probably reduces consumption; effect on prevalence uncertain	Minimal costs to health sector	Has spread rapidly among larger UK companies	Necessary to protect non-smokers; possible long term effect on prevalence
12. Paid mass media advertising campaigns	Quit rate in range 0–5%	In range $10–20 per YLS (at 2.5% quit rate)	Potentially high impact, but efficacy is controversial	High impact; potentially highly effective
C. General interventions aimed at all age groups				
13. Fiscal policy	Price elasticity about − 0.5 for consumption. Also associated with substantial falls in prevalence	No direct cost to health sector	High reach, limited only by smuggling	The single most effective measure of all: drawbacks include regressive effects on deprived groups
14. Health warnings on cigarette packets	Possibly some influence with adolescents	No direct cost	High reach	Necessary for ethical reasons
15. Product modification	Possible long term reduction in disease	Minimal costs	High reach	Desirable; ultimately limited by smokers' tastes
16. Bans on all forms of advertising	Probable effects on adult consumption and teenage prevalence	No direct costs	High reach	Desirable for many reasons, but a one-off intervention only
17. Media advocacy and creation of unpaid publicity	Elasticity of − 0.5 for consumption; linked with major declines in prevalence. Major effect is on public opinion	Cheaper than paid advertising but requires substantial resources. No Smoking Day costs $8–36 per YLS	High reach	Strongly recommended for its direct effects alone. Influence on climate of public opinion provides the essential foundation for the entire campaign

However, under the favourable conditions required for internal validity, school programmes which include training in refusal skills and related psychosocial factors, can delay recruitment to smoking for several years, but not indefinitely[6]. They are most effective at age 12–14 years, just before the period of maximum recruitment to smoking, since they have no effect on established smokers[6].

However, under real life conditions, it has proved impossible to replicate the encouraging results from pilot trials[6]. The more effective programmes are also difficult to implement as intended owing to lack of sufficient curriculum time, so that their reach is limited[6]. Although costs to the health sector are usually small, and programmes for younger children may have a possible favourable effect on parental smoking[6], the overall contribution of school programmes is relatively limited.

Other interpersonal interventions for youth

Bans on smoking by teachers and students on school premises have been implemented in a number of UK schools, though the effect on teenage prevalence is not clear[6]. Nevertheless, the education sector should be encouraged to set an example as an entirely smoke-free zone, especially as costs to the health sector are minimal.

UK trials of 'Smoke Busters' clubs for non-smoking 10–14 year-olds suggest that membership may have a possible delaying effect on recruitment to smoking, lasting for 2–3 years at most[6]. A high profile club can generate valuable publicity, but as they are costly to service, media coverage is probably the only justification for health sector funding[6]. Cessation programmes for teenagers have so far had little impact because of poor reach and low efficacy – probably owing to the fundamental instability of teenage smoking as a habit[6].

Mass media campaigns aimed mainly at youth

In a controlled trial in Vermont (USA), a combined mass media and school curriculum intervention achieved up to 40% reduction in prevalence at age 15–17 years, compared to school curriculum only. The effects lasted for at least two years after the intervention was complete[6]. However, more comprehensive programmes (though with a smaller per caput budget) comprising mass campaigns and other interventions for youth, had no effect on teenage prevalence in Minnesota or England, during a period when adult prevalence in England fell from 35% to 28%[6]. While mass campaigns can reach at least 90% of the target audience within a few months, their cost-effectiveness is relatively low – for example, the Vermont media component alone cost in the range £155 – 755 ($233 – $1135) per 'delayed smoker'[8]. Given the lack of a clear effect in Minnesota and England, mass campaigns aimed specifically at youth are unlikely to be a cost-effective investment, relative to alternative uses for the same funds.

Restrictions on sales to teenagers

Sales to children under 16 are illegal in the UK and many other countries. However, the legislation is widely ignored, so that effectiveness depends largely on the extent of compliance by shopkeepers[6]. Educational campaigns and the use of under age children to attempt supervised trial purchases, have reduced illegal sales in some locations, at minimal cost to the health sector[6].

However, despite extensive national and local activity, overall ease of purchase by minors in the UK has changed little since 1986[6]. Furthermore, since sales to mature children aged 14–16 are difficult to prevent, this intervention will have only a delaying effect at best – though it can be a source of valuable publicity[6].

Prevention: conclusions

Interventions aimed specifically at youth are, therefore, unlikely to make a major contribution to the achievement of national targets. The more effective measures are difficult to implement on a large scale, and generally have a delaying effect only. Delay does, however, result in gains to health because later starters may quit earlier, and so are at reduced risk from smoking related disease[6].

Cessation: interventions aimed at adult smokers

At any given time, 6 million (40%) (both men and women equally[9]) of the UK's 15 million smokers are contemplating quitting; of these, 2 million are actively preparing[10], and 11 million have already given up[3]. The commonest reasons cited for trying to give up are: health (87% of current or ex-smokers), expense (51%), and family pressure (43%)[3].

Interventions to promote cessation include person to person ('interpersonal') advice, either direct to the general public, or to patients in a health setting. Population level methods include restrictions on smoking in public, and the use of mass communications or health promoting policies, e.g. fiscal policy.

Interpersonal advice

Advice to the general public The provision of advice to small groups of smokers in specially organised 'smokers' advice clinics' is a relatively effective intervention, resulting in one year quit rates in the range 10–25%. However, since they are not popular with smokers, their impact is limited by low reach[3]; they are also less cost-effective than other interventions[3]. Nevertheless, they have been recommended for heavily addicted smokers[11], and they can add a positive tone to a mass campaign[3].

Advice can also be given to smokers via telephone 'quit lines', using taped messages only (a low cost, low efficacy option) or live operators (high cost, high efficacy). Reach depends on the cost to the smoker and the extent to which the number is advertised. A free quit line in Scotland staffed by counsellors and promoted as part of a mass campaign was called by 80,000 smokers, or 6% of all Scottish adult smokers, in 1992/3. After six months, 19% were non-smokers[12]; the combined cost of the campaign and phone lines was about £100 (US$150) per quitter[13].

Advice from health professionals Brief advice from a family doctor (general practitioner or GP) to smokers during routine consultations can result in up to 5% of smokers quitting [3,14]. Longer and more elaborate interventions by GPs achieve a higher quit rate, but are less cost effective[8].

Since 70% of UK adults consult their GP annually, the potential reach of brief advice is considerable. If every smoker was advised to quit at each consultation, up to 500,000, or 3% of the total, might give up each year. However, in practice, only 1 in 4 UK smokers report receiving advice from their doctor[3], and only 7% report that the doctor's advice helped them to stop[10]. There are many reasons why the theoretically high reach of brief advice is unlikely to be achieved in practice[15,16].

Nicotine replacement therapy, particularly the nicotine patch, can significantly enhance the effectiveness of GP advice, especially with more addicted smokers[17]. However, patches are less cost-effective than brief advice, both to the GP and the smoker[8].

Population level interventions

Promotion of restrictions on smoking in public In the UK and elsewhere, restrictions on smoking in public have been introduced to protect non-smokers from the effects of environmental tobacco smoke (ETS). In workplaces, this usually leads to reduced exposure to ETS and in most cases to a net fall in consumption, in the range 2–3 fewer cigarettes daily[3].

The effects on prevalence are less clear. In California, there is an association between restrictions and lower prevalence[18], but the direction of causality is not clear[3]. Only 16% of British current or ex-smokers cite workplace restrictions as a reason for trying to quit[3]. However, a fall in prevalence can be expected where employers offer cessation courses to facilitate the introduction of restrictions[19].

Costs are largely borne by employers, and implementation is rapid when publicity on the effects of ETS is combined with appropriate legislation[5], as in the UK[3]. The proportion of larger UK companies with restrictive policies rose from 6% to 80% between 1980 and 1990[3].

However, the introduction of restrictions alone is unlikely to achieve rapid declines in prevalence, though they probably have a valuable long term influence[3].

Paid mass media advertising Controlled trials suggest that mass campaigns can cause up to 5% of smokers to quit, though this finding remains controversial[3]. However, large scale paid media campaigns have been associated with rapid, major declines in prevalence, e.g. in the USA (1967–70) and Australia (1983–86)[3] as shown in Figure 1. In California, the launch of a major TV campaign in 1990 was associated with a sharp

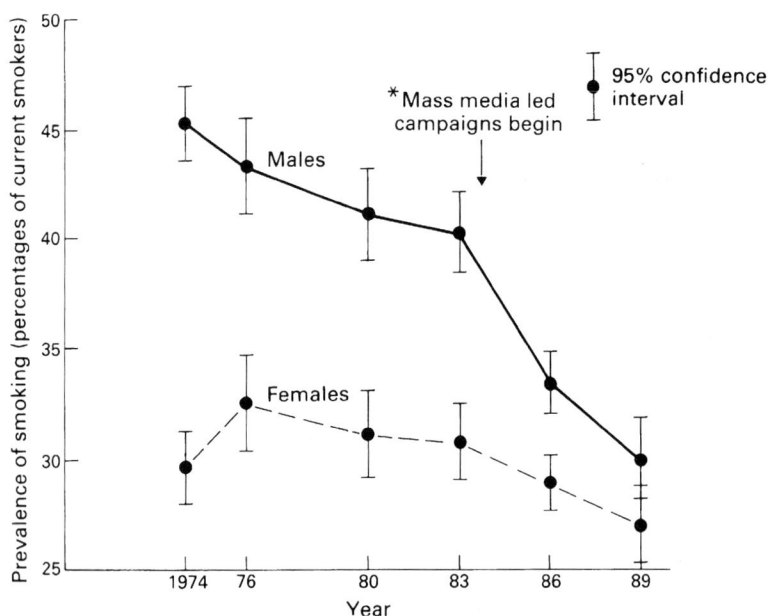

Fig. 1 Prevalence of cigarette smoking in adults aged 16 or over in Australia, 1974–89. Caption (*) added by author. Copyright © The *Medical Journal of Australia* 1991; **154**: 797–801. Reprinted with permission.

increase in reported attempts to quit[20] and a significant decline in consumption, which ceased when the campaign was temporarily interrupted[21].

Mass campaigns involving TV can reach 90% of the target audience within a few weeks; consequently, despite the large budgets required, they may still be cost-effective. In the UK, a full weight national campaign would cost at least £12 ($18) million annually[3]. If 2.5% (or 350,000) smokers quit as a result, the costs per year of life saved would be in the range £6–12 ($10–20), about the same as brief advice from a GP[8].

Interventions during pregnancy Only 55% of UK women report receiving advice to stop during pregnancy, and the resulting success rate is only in the range 5–12%[22], the majority of whom relapse after giving birth[8]. A low budget UK mass campaign had no discernible effect on prevalence among pregnant smokers[23].

Advice to pregnant smokers from health professionals is a relatively high reach, low cost intervention. It is highly cost-effective insofar as it saves the health costs required for the care of smokers' low birthweight children[8]. Further investment is therefore fully justified though, in the long run, broader actions to discourage smoking in the community generally may have greater and more lasting effects.

General interventions for all age groups

Fiscal policy

The extent to which smokers can afford to purchase cigarettes ('affordability') has a major influence on consumption (see Townsend, this issue). For every 1% increase in real price, per caput consumption typically falls by about 0.5%, both among adults and youth, provided real disposable income remains constant[3,6]. In the UK, the effect is inversely related to socioeconomic status, so wealthier smokers are less affected[24].

Not surprisingly, a sharp decline in affordability from 1980–82 was associated with one of the fastest declines in prevalence and consumption ever seen in the UK (Fig. 2) – especially among manual workers[25].

The scope for increasing taxes may ultimately be limited by smuggling and by concern for its effects on disadvantaged groups[26]. However, since higher taxes increase government revenues at no direct cost to the health sector, this is a highly cost-effective option, which achieves immediate universal reach.

Prevalence of cigarette smoking in
adults 16 and over in Great Britain
1950 - 1992

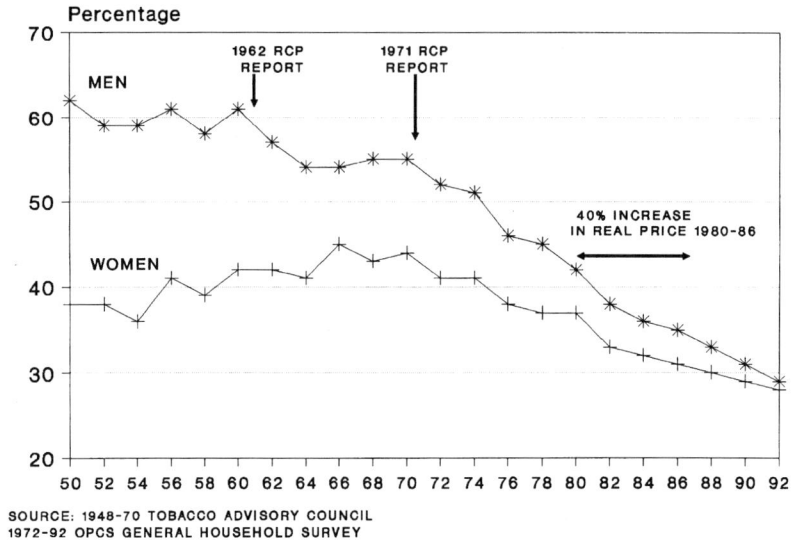

Fig. 2 Prevalence of cigarette smoking in adults 16 and over in Great Britain, 1950–92. Source: 1948–70 Tobacco Advisory Council, 1972–92 OPCS General Household Survey.

Health warnings

In many countries, health warnings on cigarette packets are compulsory, chiefly for ethical reasons, since their efficacy is limited. Adult smokers are probably little affected by them, but adolescents may be more attentive, especially to rotating, meaningful messages, which may also help to diminish the impact of cigarette advertising[27,28].

Product modification

A programme to reduce the permitted levels of tar and nicotine in tobacco products probably results in some overall gain to health, though any benefits are trivial compared to cessation[5]. The scope for increasing reductions is ultimately limited by consumer resistance and compensatory smoking behaviour[5].

Bans on all forms of cigarette advertising and promotion

In many countries, the advertising and promotion of cigarettes, etc., is either banned (e.g. Finland) or restricted (UK). Advertising definitely influences teenage attitudes, and probably their behaviour also, as well as increasing overall consumption[6].

A ban is therefore a high reach intervention, implemented at no direct cost to the health sector, and so highly cost-effective. For full efficacy, it should be linked with a requirement to package cigarettes in dull 'generic' packaging[6]. However, it is a 'one-off' intervention only, whose achievement can be counterproductive if it results in a diminution of support for more effective measures, such as fiscal policy[6].

Mass communications: creation of unpaid publicity

The health sector can make effective use of the mass media by stimulating unpaid coverage of issues related to tobacco control. This can have beneficial effects both on the behaviour of smokers and on the climate of public opinion.

Direct effects on smokers' behaviour   Almost 60% of UK ex-smokers report that they gave up without the use of any special method or advice[10]; and 87% cite health as a reason for quitting[3]. It is, therefore, not surprising that large scale media coverage of the links between smoking and health is often associated with sharp declines in the habit. For example, the publication of the 1962 and 1971 reports of the Royal College of Physicians of London on the health effects of smoking was the prime cause of the 30% decline in UK male prevalence from 1962–1980 (Fig. 2) during a period of declining real price[3]. Major bursts of health publicity may have an elasticity of response of up to −0.050, i.e. they reduce per caput consumption of cigarettes by up to 5%[29].

For this reason, the UK national health education agencies regularly publish data on smoking and health[30], and support the annual No Smoking Day (NSD), an event originally created purely to obtain unpaid media coverage. Up to 2 million smokers annually report that participation in NSD helps them to reduce smoking at least temporarily; of these, up to 45,000 (0.3% of all UK smokers) may still be abstinent one year later[3]. In the USA, a week-long series of cessation advice articles in a local newspaper, had an impact equivalent to that of 380 smokers' cessation clinics, or 1900 GPs each seeing an average of 5 smokers weekly[3].

Televised cessation advice programmes can have effects comparable to a major paid advertising campaign – though at trivial cost to the health sector[3]. Smokers' 'Quit & Win' competitions have high efficacy, but generally low impact owing to poor recruitment. However, they can also be a source of highly positive publicity[3].

Effects on public opinion Much the most important reason for creating media publicity lies in its influence on public opinion and so, ultimately, on government policy. In the UK, as elsewhere, the major components of an effective tobacco control strategy require either government funding (e.g. major health education programmes) or government support (e.g. fiscal policy).

Despite the evident efficacy of these measures, most politicians require evidence of popular support before taking action. Fortunately, studies in communications theory indicate that news stories can have measurable effects both on public opinion and on elected politicians[6]. Absence of media pressure on politicians has been cited as a prime cause for the disappointing trends in Finnish prevalence in the 1980s[6].

The costs of creating unpaid publicity are considerably lower than paid mass campaigns, but are not negligible. For example, No Smoking Day costs about £0.01 ($0.02) per head of total population annually in the UK[3,6]. An effective strategic programme to advance public policy initiatives through the media ('media advocacy'[31]) ideally requires an annual investment of at least £100,000 ($150,000) for a population of about 50 million. However, the reach of unpaid publicity is very high: over 90% of UK smokers are aware of No Smoking Day each year[3]; its cost-effectiveness is comparable to brief advice from a GP[8].

Discussion and conclusions

Despite the overall success of the UK tobacco control strategy, smoking is now a major cause of inequalities in health in the UK[26]. This is because unpaid publicity has less effect on disadvantaged groups[24], though this is probably chiefly due to the printed media rather than television[32]. Favourable fiscal policy has the opposite effect, so tending to reduce inequalities[24,26].

In view of the relative ineffectiveness of interventions aimed at youth, resources should be concentrated either on measures to promote cessation or on broader actions such as fiscal policy or an advertising ban[3]. The campaign should be supported by the setting up of a national organisation to co-ordinate activity and to act as a focus for communicating with the media, such as the UK's Action on Smoking and Health (ASH).

Although this review has considered each intervention in isolation, best results are obviously obtained when a range of actions are implemented simultaneously[33]. High reach interventions such as fiscal policy and mass communications are more likely to generate synergistic interactions than low reach activities such as interpersonal advice.

Fiscal policy and unpaid media coverage together account for the bulk of the UK decline in prevalence since 1960[3]; while fiscal policy is the most effective intervention available, its use is dependent on media advocacy to achieve the necessary public support for its implementation.

Given the respect in which health professionals, especially doctors, are held by the public, they may therefore achieve more for their patients through the media than by giving personal advice[16]. The health sector should therefore give priority to the development of a well resourced communications strategy, including funding for media training for doctors[34], since 'the best way to fight lung cancer is with a press conference'[3].

Acknowledgements

Thanks to the *Medical Journal of Australia* for permission to reproduce Figure 1, to Hilary Whent for Figure 2 and Rodney Amis for literature retrieval.

References

1 Lopez AD, Collishaw NE, Piha T. A descriptive model of the cigarette epidemic in developed countries. *Tobacco Control* 1994; 3: 242–7

2 Department of Health. *The Health of the Nation: a Strategy for Health in England.* London: HMSO, 1992

3 Reid DJ, Killoran AJ, McNeill AD, Chambers JS. Choosing the most effective health promotion options for reducing a nation's smoking prevalence. *Tobacco Control* 1992; 1: 185–97

4 An international strategy for tobacco control. *Tobacco Control* 1994; 3: 304

5 Roemer R. *Legislative Action to combat the World Tobacco Epidemic* 2nd edn. Geneva: World Health Organization, 1993

6 Reid DJ, McNeill AD, Glynn TJ. Reducing the prevalence of smoking in youth in Western countries: an international review. *Tobacco Control* 1995; 4: 266–77

7 Bruvold WH. A meta-analysis of adolescent smoking prevention programs. *Am J Public Health* 1993; 83: 872–80

8 Buck D, Godfrey C. *Helping smokers give up – guidance for purchasers on cost effectiveness.* London: York University Centre for Health Promotion, for the Health Education Authority, 1994

9 Jarvis MJ. Gender differences in smoking cessation: real or a myth? *Tobacco Control* 1994; 3: 324–8

10 West R. *Escaping the Nicotine Trap: A report on smoking cessation in the UK.* London: No Smoking Day Committee, Hamilton House, Mabledon Place, London WC1H 9TX, UK; 1995

11 Fisher EB, Lichtenstein E, Haire-Joshu D, Morgan GD, Rehberg HR. Methods, successes, and failures of smoking cessation programs. *Annu Rev Med* 1993; 44: 481–513

12 Donnan PR, Watson J, Platt S, Tannahill A, Raymond M. Predictors of successful quitting: findings from a six-month evaluation of the Smokeline campaign. *J Smoking Related Dis* 1994: 5 (suppl 1); 271–6

13 Platt S. *Evaluation of the General Public Anti-smoking Campaign: Report on the First Year (Oct 1992–Oct 1993).* Edinburgh: Health Education Board for Scotland, 1994

14 Austoker JA, Sanders D, Fowler G. Smoking and cancer: smoking cessation. *BMJ* 1994; **308**: 1478–82

15 Richmond RL, Anderson P. Research in general practice for smokers and excessive drinkers in Australia and the UK. III. Dissemination of interventions. *Addiction* 1994; **89**: 49–62

16 Chapman S. The role of doctors in promoting cessation. *BMJ* 1993; **307**: 518–19

17 Silagy C, Mant D, Fowler G, Lodge M. Meta-analysis on efficacy of nicotine replacement therapies in smoking cessation. *Lancet* 1994; **343**: 139–42

18 Woodruff TH, Rosbrook B, Pierce J, Glantz SA. Lower levels of cigarette consumption found in smoke-free workplaces in California. *Arch Intern Med* 1993; **153**: 1485–93

19 Fisher KJ, Glasgow RE, Terborg JR. Work site smoking cessation: a meta-analysis of long-term quit rates from controlled studies. *J Occup Med* 1990; **32**: 429–39

20 Popham WJ, Potter LD, Bal DG, Johnson MD, Duerr JM, Quinn V. Do anti-smoking media campaigns help smokers quit? *Public Health Rep* 1993; **108**: 510–13

21 Reid DJ. Is health education effective? In: *Health Promotion Today*. London, Health Education Authority, 1995

22 Jones K, McLeod Clark J. *A review of effective interventions in smoking and pregnancy*. London: Health Education Authority, 1993

23 Campion P, Owen L, McNeill A, McGuire C. Evaluation of a mass media campaign on smoking and pregnancy. *Addiction* 1994; **89**: 1245–54

24 Townsend J, Roderick P, Cooper J. Cigarette smoking by socioeconomic group, sex and age: effects of price, income, and health publicity. *BMJ* 1994; **309**: 923–7

25 Walters R, Whent H. *Health Update 2: Smoking* 2nd edn. London: Health Education Authority, 1995

26 Townsend J. The burden of smoking. In: Benzeval M, Judge K, Whitehead M. eds. *Tackling Inequalities in Health*. London: The King's Fund, 1995

27 Malouff J, Schutte N, Frohardt M, Deming W, Mantelli D. Preventing smoking: evaluating the potential effectiveness of health warnings. *J Psychol* 1992; **126**: 371–83

28 Naett C, Howie C. *The labelling of Tobacco Products in the European Union*. Bruxelles: European Bureau for Action on Smoking Prevention (BASP), 1993

29 Bosanquet N, Trigg A. *A Smoke-free Europe in the Year 2000: Wishful Thinking or Realistic Strategy?* Chichester, UK: Carden Publications, 1991

30 Health Education Authority. *The Smoking Epidemic: Counting the Cost in England*. London, Health Education Authority, 1991

31 Chapman S, Lupton D. *The Fight for Public Health: Principles and Practice of Media Advocacy*. London: BMJ Publishing Group, 1994

32 Reid DJ. Effects of health publicity on prevalence of smoking. *BMJ* 1994; **309**: 1441

33 Chapman S. Unravelling gossamer with boxing gloves: problems in explaining the decline in smoking. *BMJ* 1993; **307**: 429–32

34 Raw M, McNeill A. The prevention of tobacco-related disease. *Addiction* 1994; **89**: 1505–9

The ethics of tobacco advertising and advertising bans

Simon Chapman

University Department of Community Medicine, Westmead Hospital, Westmead, NSW, Australia

In this chapter, I will examine the main ethical parameters of the arguments pertaining to the alleged 'right' to advertise tobacco products and those maintaining that it should be banned. In particular, I will explore the ethics of the adoption of 'partial' bans on tobacco advertising, since there are now few countries which do not restrict tobacco advertising in some way.

The banning of all forms of tobacco advertising and promotion has long been regarded as a central platform of comprehensive tobacco control policy. Ruth Roemer's 1993 review of the regulation of tobacco lists 27 nations which claim to have totally banned tobacco advertising, with a further 77 having some form of restriction[1]. More recently, Bulgaria, Hungary, Lithuania, Moldova, Slovakia, Ukraine and Russia have also been reported to have implemented bans.

The research and public health policy literature on tobacco advertising has burgeoned as moves to ban advertising have become increasingly contested. This literature has been recently reviewed[2-4] and its scope covers the nine areas listed below (these are referenced with particularly important examples of each).

1. Documentation and commentary on changing expenditure on tobacco advertising and promotion[5], including how this expenditure ranks with other commodity advertising.
2. Econometric research into the relationship between the volume of tobacco advertising and changes in tobacco consumption[6].
3. Research into the recognition, recall, approval of, or liking for tobacco advertising[7] and sponsorship[8], usually by children; and research into the relationship between reaction to such advertising and children's subsequent use of tobacco[9].
4. Reports of ways by which tobacco advertisers circumvent voluntary codes and legal bans and restrictions[10], including evidence for product placement in films[11] and television programs[12].
5. Studies of the relationship between tobacco advertising and the (usually reduced) coverage of smoking and health by newspapers, magazines, and other media[13].

6. Evidence and commentary on the apparent targeting of non-smokers by tobacco advertisers, especially women[14], children[15] and communities with low smoking rates[16].
7. Semiotic and other interpretive studies of tobacco advertising, examining the likely intentions of advertisers in constructing text and visual copy[17]; also qualitative audience studies examining the perceptions of target audiences of this advertising[18].
8. Studies about self-reported reasons for taking up smoking, where advertising is examined as one potential reason. Such studies are commonly promoted by the tobacco industry[19].
9. Evidence relating to the buying of political and community support from groups in receipt of tobacco sponsorship and advertising[20].

With notable exceptions[21-23], the core ethical questions at the heart of proposals to both maintain or ban tobacco advertising have been assumed rather than explicated in this literature. Supporters of tobacco advertising tend to base their support on an assumed equivalence of tobacco with all other retail products and services, allowing them to point to restrictions on the advertising of their product as discriminatory and unfair. They summarise this purported equivalence in the slogan 'if a product is legally sold, it should be legally advertised', which is examined below. Those seeking to ban tobacco advertising argue that tobacco ought not to be considered an ordinary good, but one self-evidently deserving of extraordinary regulatory attention by the state because of the burden of disease caused by tobacco use.

Ethical questions about advertising generally

Part of the debate about the ethics of tobacco advertising involves consideration of ethical questions about advertising *per se*. Advertising is the attempt by owners of goods and services to persuade current and potential consumers to continue or start purchasing. The intention of advertisers is, therefore, to portray products in ways that will maximise their desirability to potential consumers. Some commentators on the ethics of advertising have sought to draw a distinction between its informative and persuasive functions, arguing that pure 'information' in advertising (as said to be exemplified by classified advertisements and yellow page telephone directory listings) is 'moral' because it facilitates rational decision-making and choice. However, 'persuasive' advertising is argued to be unethical because, drawing on Kantian ethics, it affects consumers' 'autonomy' by convincing them to purchase goods which they do not 'need'[24]. This argument has been severely criticised as resting on a false or simplistic dichotomies of wants and needs and of information and persuasion[25]—information can be highly persuasive, and the persuasive associations lent to a product by advertising can be argued to be as much part of the true 'meaning' or reality of that product to consumers as its physical properties.

Information in tobacco advertising?

One of the cornerstones of the argument in favour of advertising generally is that advertising provides consumers with information about products and services being offered for sale. Classical economists argue that efficiency is optimised when all parties in an economic transaction have maximum information. The usual sorts of information exemplified in such arguments include price, the attributes of a product and notice of availability.

Does tobacco advertising provide such information and help facilitate choice? Mention of price is virtually absent in tobacco advertising, except at point of sale, where discounting is rampant in tobacco retailing. Descriptions of product yield attributes are common in advertising and brand naming, but these are frequently specious ('fresh'), patently subjective ('luxury', 'super'). Also, because many smokers block the tiny air vent holes with their fingers or lips, thereby greatly increasing the yields of tar and nicotine they inhale when compared to the smoking machine determined yields cited in advertising and on packs, cigarette advertising is in this respect arguably misleading[26]. The argument that tobacco advertising provides information is thus largely bankrupt when examined against actual practice.

Some have argued that so-called 'tombstone' advertising—advertising showing only the cigarette pack with the product name—ought to be considered a benign non-persuasive form of tobacco advertising which might be said to satisfy the basic criteria for 'information only' advertising. The assumption here is that tombstone advertising essentially is 'here it is!' advertising, informing consumers about the name of the brand, its packaging, the number of cigarettes in it, and sometimes the tar and nicotine yields. Putting aside manipulative efforts such as *Marlboro*'s Belgian initiative during the 1980s of putting the picture of the *Marlboro* cowboy on the pack in anticipation of overcoming a move to tombstone advertising, it is fallacious to argue that pack-only advertising is somehow devoid of persuasive intent. A great deal of research goes into the selection of names, pack design[27] and into the selection of seemingly bland words in the slogans that accompany pictures of packs. Every effort is made to make tombstone advertising as enticing as possible.

Selectivity

Because there are limits to the time or space any advertisement occupies in the media, its content cannot possibly cover all aspects of a product's qualities, its origin, its various uses, all consequences that might conceivably flow from its use and so on. Instead, advertisers **cannot avoid** being selective about what they say and infer about their products. Understandably, in needing to be selective and in intending that advertising should persuade consumers, advertisers select emphases that are predicted to make products seem desirable.

We do not expect an advertiser of cars to take up the limited advertising space and time available drawing consumers' attention to the possible adverse financial consequences of owning a car, to the statistical probabilities of car drivers being killed or injured, or to the relative merits of using public transport. Yet all of these issues are plainly relevant to car buyers. Parallel questions can be asked about advertising for any product, including tobacco. The ethical questions arising here ask whether, in the inevitable exercise of selectivity in constructing advertisements, any consumer deception is involved. Is advertising intrinsically misleading to consumers if it fails, as it always does, to fully describe every possible facet of a product and consequence of its use?

If the answer to this is yes, then such a radical standard for determining consumer deception will condemn **all** advertising as unethical and provides no insight into whether tobacco advertising is in any way exceptional, warranting the special treatment it gets.

Are tobacco advertisements lies?

Lying is *prima facie* unethical. Can it be said that tobacco advertising constitutes lying? A lie is a statement made by one who does not believe it with the intention that someone else shall be led to believe it[28]. There are three critical elements to this definition when applying it to tobacco advertising: determining what it is that tobacco advertising proposes to its audiences; establishing that tobacco advertisers know these propositions to be false; and a conception of the audience as those who believe any 'false' claims made in tobacco advertising to be true.

The first of these elements is most problematical. Most contemporary tobacco advertising makes very few written or verbal propositions about the tobacco advertised that can be simply assessed as true or false. Rather, the advertisements seek to position a set of carefully market researched associations in **apposition** to the brands being advertised in the attempt to forge positive associations about tobacco, smoking and smokers. The associations are designed to attach attributes to particular brands so that consumers will identify these brands as compatible with their desired presentation of self in everyday life, or to offer solutions to contradictions in the lives of consumers or in their feelings about smoking[17]. Here, cigarette advertisements and brand names make semiotic propositions about (for example) personal potency to the socially impotent, relaxation to the harried, a sense of modernity to those fearful of being seen as conservative, or a sense of belonging to the lonely (one Australian brand is named *Escort*, a Filipino brand *Hope*).

These are no more 'lies' or false statements than the proposition that 'Coke adds life'. These are simply commercially motivated attempts at socially constructing particular meanings for smoking or *Coca Cola*. For every person who insists that the 'real' meaning of smoking is something to do with disease and addiction, there are many who associate smoking with the meanings portrayed in tobacco advertising. It is specious to argue that one meaning is 'true' while others are false, and hence to then demonstrate that tobacco advertisers 'knew' that a suggestion in their advertising that smoking equals sophistication was false. While tobacco advertising remains a largely connotative form of communication, demonstrating that it peddles lies and demonstrable falsehoods will be difficult.

Deception through omission?

Another way of approaching the question of whether advertising is misleading is to ask whether there are aspects of a product which if **omitted** from advertising, would result in consumers being misled. For example, consumer protection laws in many countries insist that financial services advertising make explicit claims about terms of credit, so serious are the consequences for consumers should they be misled. The questions arising here concern whether there are fundamental issues about a product that should be mandatory in any advertising for it. With tobacco advertising, many argue that the risks of use are so high that, at very least, advertising should be accompanied by detailed health warnings worded so as to maximise their comprehensibility and resonance.

However, here many have pointed out the tobacco industry's long record in constructing advertising designed to mock, distract and generally undermine such health warnings. In Australia in 1995, Rothmans modified its pack design after bold new warnings were introduced[29] so that a warning on the front of the flip-top box such as 'Smoking when pregnant harms your baby' is accompanied by the contemptuous advertising slogan 'Anyhow . . . have a Winfield' printed on the inside of the flip-top box. This mockery has recently reached its apotheosis with the launch and promotion of *Death* cigarettes in the Europe[30]. Here *Death*'s owners have turned health warnings into an 'in your face' gesture of proud defiance so that the risks of smoking are not only acknowledged, but held out as a badge of audacity, risk-taking and scorn on safe living.

The advent of the *Death* brand illustrates perhaps more completely than all previous argument, the ability of advertising to appropriate virtually any appeal — even a message overtly antithetical to the product — and turn it into a marketing edge using the massive advertising budgets available to the industry. This ability would appear to transcend all guidelines and thematic restraints on advertising copy and hence act to largely neutralise the intent of health warnings for some people.

Tobacco is an extraordinary product

Some commentators have argued that the ethics of advertising should be inextricably linked to questions about the 'goodness' of the products being advertised. Leiser[31] and Lee[32] argue that 'the advertisement of a bad product cannot be good', with Leiser arguing that persuasive and seductive appeals can be ethically defensible if they have been put to the service of promoting beneficial ends (for example, using nostalgic appeals to country life to sell fruit and vegetables or using scare tactics to persuade people not to drink alcohol before driving). This emphasis on the product rather than on the way it is advertised is at the heart of all concern about tobacco advertising. Critics of the RJ Reynolds' *Joe Camel* cartoon character's appeal to very young children have not been critical of the use of an anthropomorphic cartoon character in itself (cartoons have been often used to promote health), but rather of the use of the cartoon to promote *Camel* cigarettes to children. Critics of the use of sexuality to sell cigarettes are not generally opposed to sensual or erotic imagery, but to the use to which it is put: to make cigarettes seem attractive.

Herein lies the nub of opposition to tobacco advertising. Its critics argue that whatever its effects (and using reductionist methodologies, these are extraordinarily difficult to dissect from the contemporaneous influence of other tobacco control strategies[33]) the **intention** of tobacco advertisers is by definition to promote tobacco use. The 'brand switching' argument is quite irrelevant to this concern, for a brand cannot be promoted without promoting smoking itself. If governments have policies to reduce tobacco use, policies that allow tobacco advertising are simply inconsistent with these.

By any standard, tobacco is no ordinary product. A recent US Surgeon General stated in the preface to the 1990 Surgeon General's report on smoking: 'it is safe to say that smoking represents the most extensively documented cause of disease ever investigated in the history of biomedical research'. The first section of this book documents the effects of tobacco use still further. Efforts to ban tobacco advertising have not been mounted because of ethical concerns for the imagery and persuasive rhetoric employed, but because the intention of this advertising is to promote tobacco use. And there is a wealth of evidence that it succeeds in doing so[4].

Being no ordinary product in causing the catastrophic degree of harm and cost to both individuals and the state that it does throughout populations, advocates of banning advertising argue that it is reasonable that tobacco should be subject to extraordinary controls designed to reduce this harm. Controlling advertising is but one form of such control.

Is there a 'right' to advertise?

Defenders of tobacco advertising tend to assume a free marketing philosophy where any restrictions on advertising are seen as ethically offensive to the sovereignty of business interests. As Milton Friedman has written: 'few trends could so thoroughly undermine the very foundations of our free society as the acceptance by corporate officials of a social responsibility other than to make as much money for their shareholders as possible' [34]. However, governments intervene in marketplaces in many ways, ranging from the outright banning of products already in a marketplace (e.g. thalidomide) or of newly developed products (e.g. many instances of unsafe toys, furniture, etc.), through restrictions on sales, packaging and advertising information requirements, to restrictions and bans on advertising. At one extreme of regulation, governments frequently exercise their rights to ban products outright, typically citing consumer protection from unsafe goods as their rationale. In many countries, certain therapeutic goods are available only through registered pharmacies with consumer access requiring a doctors' prescription. In many countries, the supply of alcohol, firearms and explosives, while not illegal, is strictly regulated and conditional. In Australia, it is illegal to sell high powered motorcycles to people with (beginners') provisional licenses. Finally, in some countries drugs such as strong analgesics and bronchodilators are freely available to consumers through pharmacies, but are not permitted by law to be advertised directly to the public because of concerns that advertising may promote inappropriate use.

This range of government intervention illustrates that restrictions on advertising represent only one strategy in the attempt to control the use of products that have known potential to affect adversely either those who use them or the general public. There is no more a 'right' to advertise than there is a 'right' to sell. Both activities are frequently subsumed by broader considerations of public benefit, welfare and safety. These considerations can be paternalistic[35] (justified by concern to protect individuals from the consequences of their own behaviour, particularly when it can be demonstrated that individuals have inadequate or erroneous knowledge about the range, probability and severity of these consequences), or Millean[36] (based on concerns to restrain individual liberty if its expression has adverse consequences for others).

Some libertarians argue that paternalism is ethically unjustified—people should be free to risk harm to themselves provided that they can demonstrate that they are fully informed about the probability of, and the nature of, the harm they risk. While many people living in nations which have histories of health education about the risks of tobacco use are informed in general terms about smoking, their knowledge is often inadequate to any usual test of informed consent. This is much more the case in nations with high illiteracy rates and poor records in health education. And even if it could be established that smokers were well-informed about the risks they face, Goodin argues: 'we do not leave it to the discretion of consumers, however well-informed, whether or not to drink grossly polluted water, ingest grossly contaminated foods, or inject grossly dangerous drugs. We simply prohibit such things, on grounds of public health, by appeal to utilitarian calculations of one sort or another (p587)'[22].

No nation prohibits tobacco, and no internationally recognised public health agency has called for tobacco to be banned in the way that Goodin's argument above might imply. Almost all international public health agencies, though, have called for tobacco advertising to be banned.

The cornerstone of arguments used by proponents of the continuation of tobacco advertising is that the only factor relevant to whether a product should be advertised is its current legal status. By this argument, the industry would agree that illicit drugs should not be advertised, but would presumably (along with most in public health) support the lifting of any restrictions on the advertising of condoms. This insistence on the current legal status of tobacco is indifferent to the history of research into tobacco whereby its consequences to health only became established long after its use and manufacturing infrastructure became widespread. As many have argued, if tobacco had been recently 'invented' and subject to the tests of safety required of food and drugs, no nation would release it onto the market in the way it is sold today.

The rejoinder to this by defenders of tobacco advertising is to make hollow calls for governments to declare tobacco illegal if they are sincere in their concerns. When governments ignore such taunts, supporters of tobacco advertising allege hypocrisy on the part of governments, pointing to their appetite for tobacco excise tax.

As argued above, concern to control use of any product can be addressed through a variety of policies, of which outright banning is the furthest extreme. Considerations of proportionality—making sure that restrictions and controls imposed are no broader than necessary to achieve the desired ends — can make a decision to ban advertising while not banning the product entirely reasonable.

Is advertising 'free speech'?

Proponents of tobacco advertising have sought to argue that commercial speech is a form of free speech and, therefore, sacrosanct under constitutional guarantees in many democracies[37]. This argument has been repeatedly rejected by courts which, in the USA, have ruled on matters as diverse as casinos and commercial activities on university campuses that governments have a right to restrict commercial speech through concern about wider community issues[21].

Tobacco advertising and children

In many countries, it is illegal to sell tobacco to children. This is of critical relevance to any discussion on the ethics of tobacco advertising. Where laws forbid the sale of tobacco products to children, it is because children are said to be below an age where their informed consent can be assumed. It is, therefore, reasoned that tobacco advertising appeals directed at them or which can be shown to appeal to them are unethical in that they seek or cause to influence consent in people deemed legally incapable of consenting.

It has been repeatedly shown that children do indeed see, recall, admire, discuss and generally relate to advertising in the same sort of ways that adults are intended to do by tobacco advertisers. Apart from the obvious point that the tobacco industry makes much money from sales to underage smokers[38], the research on the impact of advertising on children makes nonsense of any pretence that advertising is 'targeted' only to adult smokers.

With the exception of premises where children are forbidden by law from entering (for example casinos, legal brothels, some premises licensed to sell alcohol), there are no advertising sites nor media to which children do not have the same access as adults. Some countries have arrangements, usually in the form of voluntary codes negotiated with the tobacco industry, that tobacco advertising will be 'restrained' in various ways. In entering such voluntary agreements, the tobacco industry typically asserts that it is not intent on targeting its advertising at children, further asserting that it regards smoking as 'an adult custom' and does not wish children to smoke.

For example, several countries in the past have endorsed voluntary agreements with the industry whereby cigarette advertisements will only be screened on television late at night, and not placed on billboards closer than 200 metres from schools. In such arrangements, an admission is being made by government and industry, as parties to these agreements, that there is a case for trying to minimise the exposure of children to such advertising — that if they were exposed, the advertisements might succeed in the same intent that they have for adults.

In practice, the logic of partial or selective tobacco advertising bans is equivalent to the ambition to be 'a little bit pregnant'. Many children do not go to bed before the arbitrary times after which cigarette advertising is screened, and with the popularisation of video recorders, many children record programs including advertisements screened after their bedtime. The logic of banning tobacco billboards adjacent to schools is even more absurd. Here, it is being suggested that a child sighting such a billboard 195 metres from a school might be influenced by its message, but the same child sighting the same advertisement 205 metres from a school would somehow be immune from its persuasions.

Partial bans carry with them an ethical conviction that tobacco advertising should be controlled, but belie this conviction by allowing the very same advertising that is banned to be displayed in the different media still permitted to carry such advertising. Such absurdity can only be interpreted as the product of an ethical duplicity cynically put to the service of collusive governmental and industry posturing about their responsibilities to children.

References

1 Roemer R. *Legislative action to combat the world tobacco epidemic.* 2nd edn. Geneva: World Health Organization, 1993
2 Toxic Substances Board. *Health or tobacco: an end to tobacco advertising and promotion.* Wellington, New Zealand: May 1989
3 Smee C. *Effect of tobacco advertising on tobacco consumption: a discussion document reviewing the evidence.* Department of Health, UK; 1992
4 US Surgeon General. *Preventing tobacco use among young people.* US Department of Health and Human Services, Public Health Service, Centers for Disease Control, Center for Health Promotion and Education, Office on Smoking and Health. Rockville, MD: 1994
5 Federal Trade Commission. Cigarette advertising and promotion in the United States, 1992. *Tobacco Control* 1994; **3**: 286–9
6 Laugesen M, Meads C. Tobacco advertising restrictions, price, income and tobacco consumption in OECD countries, 1960–1986. *Br J Addict* 1991; **86**: 1343–54
7 Aitken PP, Leathar DS, O'Hagan FJ, Squair SI. Children's awareness of cigarette advertisements and brand imagery. *Br J Addict* 1987; **82**: 615–22
8 Aitken PP, Leathar DS, Squair SI. Children's awareness of cigarette brand sponsorship of sports and games in the UK. *Health Ed Res* 1986; **1**: 203–11
9 Botvin GJ, Goldberg CJ, Botvin EM, Dusenbury L. Smoking behavior of adolescents exposed to cigarette advertising. *Public Health Rep* 1993; **108**: 217–24
10 Blum A. The Marlboro Grand Prix: circumvention of the television ban on tobacco advertising. *N Engl J Med* 1991; **324**: 913–17

11 Hazan AR, Lipton HL, Glantz SA. Popular films do not reflect current tobacco use. *Am J Public Health* 1994; **84**: 998–1000

12 Hazan AR, Glantz SA. Current trends in tobacco use on prime-time fictional television. *Am J Public Health* 1995; **85**: 116–17

13 Warner KE, Goldenhar LM, McLaughlin CG. Cigarette advertising and magazine coverage of the hazards of smoking: a statistical analysis. *N Engl J Med* 1992; **326**: 305–9

14 Ernster VL. Women, smoking, cigarette advertising and cancer. Special issue: women and cancer. *Women Health* 1986; **11**: 217–35

15 Fischer PM, Schwartz MP, Richards JW, Goldstein AO, Rojas TH. Brand logo recognition by children aged 3 to 6 years. Mickey Mouse and Old Joe the Camel. *JAMA* 1991; **266**: 3145–8

16 Kawane H. Smoking among women in Japan. *Lancet* 1991; **337**: 851

17 Chapman S. *Great expectorations: advertising and the tobacco industry.* London: Comedia, 1986

18 Hastings GB, Ryan H, Teer P, MacKintosh AM. Cigarette advertising and children's smoking: why Reg was withdrawn. *BMJ* 1994; **309**: 933–7

19 Pollay RW. Pertinent research and impertinent opinions: our contributions to the cigarette advertising policy debate. *J Advertising* 1993; **22**: 110–17

20 Robinson RG, Barry M, Bloch M *et al*. Report of the Tobacco Policy Research Group on marketing and promotion targeted at African-Americans, Latinos and women. *Tobacco Control* 1992; **4** (Suppl.)

21 Gostin LO, Brandt AM. Criteria for evaluating a ban on the advertisement of cigarettes. *JAMA* 1993; **269**: 904–9

22 Goodin RE. The ethics of smoking. *Ethics* 1989; **99**: 574–624

23 Quinn JF. Moral theory and defective tobacco advertising and warnings. (The business ethics of Cipollone versus Liggett Group). *J Bus Ethics* 1989; **8**: 831–40

24 Santilli PC. The informative and persuasive functions of advertising: a moral appraisal. *J Bus Ethics* 1983; **2**: 27–34

25 Emamalizadeh H. The informative and persuasive functions of advertising: a moral appraisal — a comment. *J Bus Ethics* 1985; **4**: 151–3

26 Kozlowski LT, Pillitteri JL, Sweeney CT. Misuse of 'light' cigarettes by means of vent blocking. *J Subst Abuse* 1994; **6**: 333–6

27 Cunningham R, Kyle K. The case for plain packaging. *Tobacco Control* 1995; **4**: 80–6

28 Isenberg A. Conditions for lying. In: Beauchamp TL, Bowie NE. eds. *Ethical theory and business.* Englewood Cliffs, NJ: Prentice-Hall 1983: pp 316–18

29 Chapman S. Industry down again down under. *Tobacco Control* 1995; **4**: 17–18

30 Anon. Enlightenment on the road to death. *Lancet* 1994; **343**: 1109–10

31 Leiser BM. Beyond fraud and deception: the moral uses of advertising. In: Donaldson T, Wehane PH. eds. *Ethical issues in business.* Englewood Cliffs, NJ: Prentice-Hall, 1979 pp59–66,

32 Lee K-H. The informative and persuasive functions of advertising: a moral appraisal — a further comment. *J Bus Ethics* 1987; **6**: 55–7

33 Chapman S. Unravelling gossamer with boxing gloves: problems in explaining the decline in smoking. *BMJ* 1993; **307**: 429–32

34 Friedman M, Friedman RD. Capitalism and freedom. Chicago: University of Chicago, 1962

35 Dworkin G. Paternalism. *Monist* 1983; **56**: 64–84

36 Mill JS. On liberty. (1859) In: Wollheim R. ed. *Three essays.* Oxford: Oxford University Press, 1975, pp 1–141

37 Luik JC. ed. *Freedom of expression. The case against tobacco advertising bans.* Catharines, Ontario: Gray Matters Press, 1991

38 Girgis A, Doran CM, Sanson-Fisher RW, Walsh RA. Smoking by adolescents: large revenue but little for prevention. *Aust J Public Health* 1995; **19**: 29–33

Price and consumption of tobacco

Joy Townsend

MRC Epidemiology and Medical Care Unit, Wolfson Institute of Preventive Medicine, The Medical College of St Bartholomew's Hospital, London, UK

Progressive increases in cigarette tax rates provide a powerful contribution to policy for reducing cigarette consumption and generate extra government revenue. The policy has been most effective in groups for whom health publicity effects have been least so, but special provision may be necessary to avoid hardship to poor families.

In the seventeenth century, James I of England initiated probably the first 'tax for health reasons' and raised tobacco tax 40-fold from 2 to 82 pence per pound, making tobacco more expensive than silver. Currently tobacco is again a cheap product; even in countries where the price is relatively high, a cigarette will cost considerably less then a snack item or a drink, so smokers can afford not the odd one or two, but usually 20 or so a day. This is the major health problem of cigarettes. This chapter will consider the impact of changes in tobacco prices on different groups of smokers, as well as the political and social implications.

As an illustration of smokers' response to price changes, Figure 1 shows how cigarette consumption has varied inversely with the real price of cigarettes in the UK over the last quarter of a century[1]. It is apparent that smoking increased during periods when the price of cigarettes fell in real terms, during the early 1970s and late 1980s, and fell when real cigarette prices rose in the mid-1970s and during the early 1980s and 1990s. Similar counter movements of smoking with relative cigarette price have been shown for several countries including France[2], Canada[3] and South Africa[4].

Price (or income) elasticity of demand is the usual measure of responsiveness to changes in real price of cigarettes (or real income). It is unit free and is defined as the percentage change in consumption for each 1% change in price (or income), usually adjusted for the rate of inflation. Elasticities of demand for cigarettes or tobacco, have been assessed for many countries over several time periods using a variety of econometric models. Estimates have varied between about -0.2 and -0.9 and have clustered about -0.5 (Table 1) (the negative sign denotes the negative relationship between price and demand). This suggests that, on average, cigarette consumption reduces by about 0.5% for every 1% increase in its real price. Few studies, apart from some for specific subsets

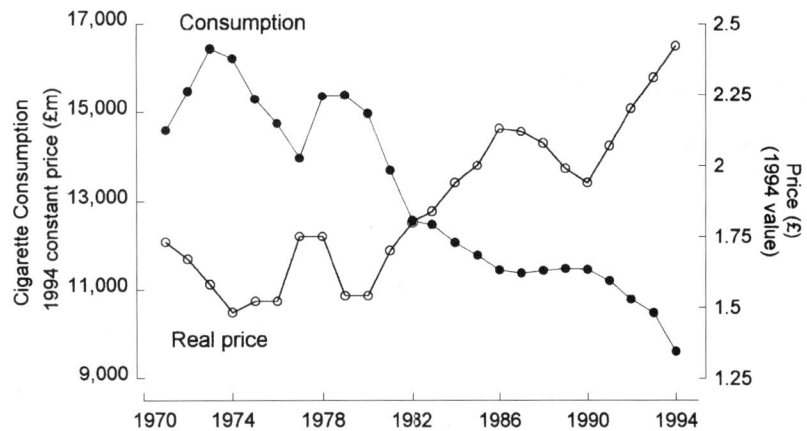

Fig. 1 The relationship between the price of cigarettes and consumption, 1971–94. Both variables are adjusted for inflation.

of smokers, report significantly different values. Estimates have been surprisingly robust over time, place and price level, being higher mostly for periods of rapid price increase, and lower for countries with relatively low tobacco prices and high incomes such as the USA. There seems to be some indication from USA, Ireland and the UK that price elasticities have fallen slightly over time, possibly due to rising income levels[5]. Higher price responses have been reported for lower income and socioeconomic groups and possibly for teenagers as will be discussed later.

Table 1 Estimates of price and income elasticities of demand for cigarettes

Study	Data	Price elasticity	Income elasticity
Andrews & Franke (1991)[5]	Meta-analysis		
UK		−0.5	0.4
US		−0.7	0.5
Other		−0.7	0.4
Post 1970		−0.4	0.3
Townsend (1988)[15]	Europe 1986–88	−0.4	0.5
Chapman & Richardson*	New Guinea 1973–86	−0.7	0.9
Worgotter & Kunze (1986)*	Austria 1955–83	−0.5	
Walsh (1980)*	Ireland post 1961	−0.4	

*Cited in Andrews & Franke (1991)[5]

Price effects by age

The price response of young smokers and young potential smokers is of particular interest, as this is the age of recruitment to smoking and there has been an apparent lack of success of health education in reducing teenage smoking. Lewit and Coate[6] studied teenage smoking in the USA and concluded that teenagers are highly responsive to cigarette prices (elasticity −1.4). There is now differing evidence from the USA suggesting a much lower price elasticity among teenagers, not significantly different from the estimate of −0.23 for American adults[7]. A UK study of smoking during 1972–90, reported[8] that the most price sensitive smokers were women, and men aged 25–60 years. Young men, on the other hand, were more influenced by income than price, showing a high response to income changes and a non-significant response to price. Young people generally have relatively low incomes with a high proportion available for discretionary expenditure, so changes in income are likely to have relatively greater effect on their smoking patterns. These results do not confirm the findings of Lewit and Coate and are more compatible with the more recent results for the USA. They do, however, suggest that cigarette consumption in teenage women may be significantly affected by price rises, although for them the effects of price and income appear to be interrelated. There will be an indirect longer term price influence also via effects on parents, as it is well established that the probability of a young person becoming a regular smoker is positively related to parental smoking.

Price effects by socioeconomic group

Tobacco price and taxation are likely to have different effects on different income and socioeconomic groups. Low income groups tend to smoke more, but reduce their smoking more in response to tax increases. Conversely, they are more likely to be encouraged to smoke by a reduction in the real price. The above UK analysis of cigarette consumption reported[8] that men and women in socioeconomic group (SEG) 1 and 2 (professional workers, managers and their wives) did not respond to changes in cigarette price, whereas adults in SEGs 3 and 4 (clerical workers, skilled and semi-skilled manual workers) responded in the middle range with a price elasticity of about −0.5 to −0.7. Unskilled manual workers and their wives (SEG 5) showed the highest response with elasticities of −1.0 for men and −0.9 for women (Table 2).

There has been much debate about whether cigarette price affects the prevalence of smoking as well as the average adult consumption. The recent UK analysis[8] reported significant elasticities of prevalence of −0.6 for men in socioeconomic group 5 (unskilled manual workers), −0.23 for all women and −0.5 for women in socioeconomic group 5. These are important results as socioeconomic group 5 is the group for whom prevalence of smoking is highest, and for whom health education has been least effective.

Table 2   Price elasticities by socioeconomic group[8] and income[10]

	Price elasticity	Health publicity effect
Men SEG		
1 (Professional)	0.0	−4.5% p.a.***
2 (Managerial)	−0.1	−3.5% p.a.***
3 (Clerical)	−0.7*	−3.0% p.a.*
3 (Skilled manual)	−0.5*	−2.0% p.a.**
4 (Semi-skilled manual)	−0.5*	−1.5% p.a.**
5 (Unskilled manual)	−1.0*	0% p.a.
Women SEG		
1 (Professional)	0.5	−3.0% p.a.**
2 (Managerial)	−0.3	−2.5% p.a.***
3 (Clerical)	−0.7**	−1.0% p.a.
3 (Skilled manual)	−0.7*	−0.5% p.a.
4 (Semi-skilled manual)	−0.6*	−0.5% p.a.
5 (Unskilled manual)	−0.9*	−1.0% p.a.
Income percentile		
90–100	−0.3	
76–90	−0.4	
26–75	−0.5	
0–25	−0.6	

*$P < 0.05$; **$P < 0.01$; ***$P < 0.001$

Atkinson *et al.*[9] and Fry and Pashardes[10] have also reported significantly different responses to tobacco price in UK households with different incomes (Table 2) and by factors related to socioeconomic group, such as house ownership. There has been little work on smoking by income and socioeconomic group for other countries, and it is important that relevant data are collected, so that the impact of price changes may be more fully understood.

Cigarette prices and the *Health of the Nation* targets

Many countries have targets for indicators of the health of their citizens. The UK Government has set targets for the year 2000 for various indicators in the *Health of the Nation* report including reductions in heart disease and cancer mortality[11]. To support these and other *Health of the Nation* concerns, specific targets have been set to reduce adult smoking prevalence from about 30% in 1990 to 20% by the end of the decade, to reduce underage smoking from 8% to less than 6% of 11–15 year olds, and smoking during pregnancy so that at least one-third of smokers give up at the beginning of their pregnancy. The UK Government has committed itself to using the rate of tobacco taxation as one instrument for achieving these targets (i.e. as a sumptuary tax) by raising tax rate on cigarettes in real terms by at least 3% per annum in future budgets, thus increasing cigarette prices by about 2.5% per annum. The 23% reduction in smoking in the UK during 1976–1988 was achieved about equally (17% each) by an overall rise in cigarette prices and by health publicity[12]. These effects were reduced, however, by some 12% due to the influence on smoking of the rise in real income over the period. Predictions of the potential for different elements of smoking control policy to achieve the national targets, estimate that the combined effects of an advertising ban, sustained health promotion about tobacco, GP smoking advice to 95% of patients who smoke, good smoking control policies in public places and the work place and the effects of a modest increase in real incomes of 1.5% per annum would, on optimistic projections from present known effects, achieve at best half the reduction necessary to achieve the adult targets. The full achievement would need a considerable extra boost from the remaining policy, a 5% price rise annually above the rate of inflation[12] until the year 2000. The Government's commitment to a 3% annual tax rise would not achieve this and neither is there a full commitment to the other policies, particularly regarding a ban on advertising. Without the latter, tobacco price would need to be increased still further, probably to about 6.5% per annum until the year 2000. In fact tax rises have been above the minimum and the adult targets are on trend at present. Underage smoking prevalence, however, has not reduced towards the targets[13], and current data on smoking in pregnancy are not yet available.

Price and consumption in Europe

Cigarette prices and consumption vary within the European Union both absolutely and relative to incomes[14]. There is a 5-fold price range between 0.71 ECUs for the most popular brand of cigarettes sold in Spain to 3.60 ECUs a pack in Denmark (1 ECU is approximately £0.82 or US$1.32). If prices are standardised for cost of living, the range narrows to 4-fold. Average smoking varies from about 5 cigarettes per day per adult in The Netherlands to about twice that level in Greece. A cross sectional study of smoking and price in 27 European countries, including all EC countries, carried out for the World Health Organization, reported a price elasticity of demand for cigarettes across Europe of -0.4 and an income elasticity of demand for cigarettes of 0.5[15]. This means that cigarette consumption will rise with incomes unless there are counter policies.

The type of tobacco used also varies, with hand rolling being particularly important in The Netherlands (49% of all consumption), Denmark (27%) Belgium (21%), Germany (10%), France (5%) and UK

(4%). This is relevant to pricing policy, as in many countries (although not the UK) hand rolling materials are taxed at a significantly lower rate than are manufactured cigarettes, although, when made into hand rolled cigarettes, they often lead to higher tar yields. In some countries, significant amounts of tobacco are smoked as cigars or in pipes, or used as oral or nasal snuff. The relative prices of these alternatives and the relative associated health risks, have important implications for overall tobacco consumption and disease. It is important to have equivalent taxation of alternative tobacco products, if taxation is to be effective in reducing health risks.

Tobacco tax structure

The European Union's excise harmonization agreement set the minimum total tax on cigarettes at 70% of the retail price. This theoretically leaves member countries free to increase cigarette taxes as they wish subject to a **maximum** proportion of the tax (55%) to be raised as a 'specific' tax per cigarette in money terms, whereas the *ad valorem* element (percentage of price) may be anything up to 95% of the tax[16]. The agreement does not substantially reduce the wide range of cigarette tax levels in the European Union, and there is concern that if cross border buying is substantial, average cigarette prices will effectively fall, although this does not appear to be the case. Smuggling between high and low tax countries has not been widespread, but still presents a strong rationale for trying to harmonise taxes and prices upwards[17]. (Smuggling has been mainly of 'duty free' cigarettes from outside the European Union, and it is estimated that 30% of cigarette exports globally are illegally imported.) In the interests of public health and harmonization, the minimum tax rate needs to be raised and expressed in money terms, i.e. the specific rate, rather than *ad valorem* as at present. Whatever the tobacco tax structure in operation, the industry may try to minimise its impact. If tax is by weight of tobacco, manufacturers may try to reduce the tax per cigarette by reducing the size of each cigarette as in the UK prior to joining the European Union. If tax is per cigarette, the industry may try to reduce the impact of the tax by increasing cigarette size to king size or super kingsize. The industry has most control over tax (per cigarette or by weight) when tax is entirely or mainly levied as an *ad valorem* tax, as a high percentage of a low price will still yield a low tax, as is in evidence in Spain and much of southern Europe (Table 3). This is shown by the low prices found where this structure operates: because basic cost of tobacco is low, the price paid by consumers, even after application of a high percentage tax, is still relatively low, which encourages high tobacco

Table 3 Effects of tax structure

Tobacco tax	Effect	Public health implication
By weight of tobacco	Manufacturers reduce size of cigarette	Beneficial
By cigarette	Manufacturers increase size of cigarette	Detrimental
Specific	Manufacturers' influence limited	Beneficial if high
Per valorem	Manufacturers keep base level low	Limited benefit
Low for non cigarette products	Smokers switch to non–cigarette	Limits benefit of tax
High tax for high tar	Smokers switch to lower tar	Slightly beneficial

consumption. In the interest of health, tax should be related in some way to weight of tobacco. Policies, such as careful monitoring of imports and possibly stamping packets for country of origin and excise duty paid are needed to deter illegal trading.

Tax revenue efficiency

Governments have three reasons to raise taxes: to raise revenue; to correct for externalities, such as health costs; and to deter consumption (sumptuary tax). Tobacco tax probably fulfils all these criteria. It is in the unique position also of being a popular tax in several countries, as surveys have reported a significant part of the population in favour – even a significant minority of smokers. Tobacco tax is a relatively efficient vehicle for raising revenue as it has an elasticity of total revenue with respect to tax rate of possibly 0.6–0.9 in the UK compared with 0.2 for spirits and 0.6 for wine[18]. This means that a 1% increase in tobacco tax results in about a 0.6–0.9% increase in tax revenue. This is demonstrated in Figure 2 which shows how real value of tobacco tax revenue has risen and fallen with changes in real cigarette price (determined mostly by tax) in the UK 1971–93 and demonstrates that tax revenue not only rises with tax rises but falls dramatically if tax does not keep up with inflation.

Given that a government needs revenue, the criteria for economic efficiency in taxation are, after Ramsey[19] and Baumol and Bradford[20], that they should have the effect of reducing demand for all commodities in the same proportion, should distort consumer choice as little as possible, and direct tax payers as little as possible to less preferred patterns of consumption. This efficiency criterion has sometimes been interpreted to mean that all commodities should be taxed at the same rate, but this is false for two reasons[21]. A uniform tax will distort the choice both between leisure and work and between goods with different price elasticities. If higher taxes are levied on goods with inelastic demand, which will be bought in some measure in any case, a lower rate can be levied on other goods, disincentive to work is decreased and there

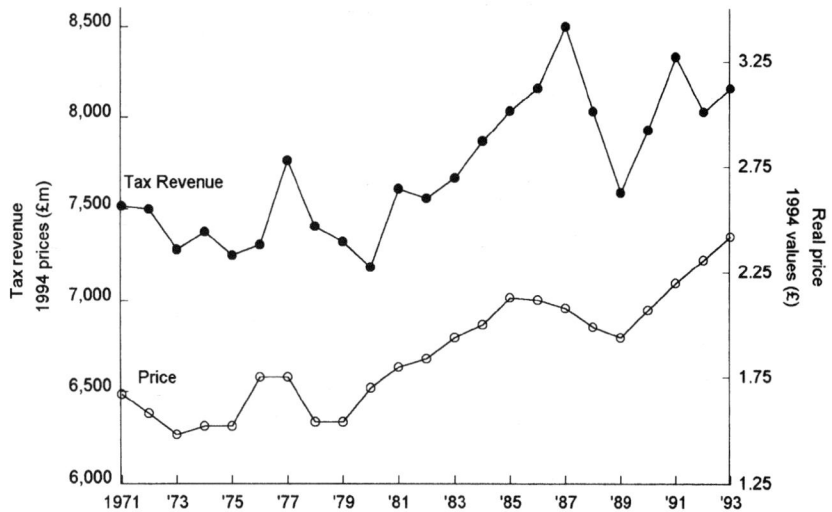

Fig. 2 The relationship between the price of cigarettes and tax revenue, 1970–93. Both variables are adjusted for inflation.

is little distortion in consumption of goods. Similarly, the argument goes, higher taxes should be imposed on goods which are substitutes for work or complements to leisure, and lighter taxes on activities which are complementary to work[21]. The related argument for higher tax on goods with relatively low price elasticity of demand, is that the dead weight welfare loss or excess burden is thus minimised[18]. (The excess burden of a tax increase is the consumers' loss of utility [roughly satisfaction] from buying less of the product at the higher price, minus the gain to the government in tax revenue. It can be expressed as a percentage of the tax revenue from the tax increase. For tobacco, the percentage excess burden is relatively low at 17%[18] compared, for example, with 500% for spirits. This means that £100 extra tax revenue would cost supposedly £117 in 'lost satisfaction' to the smoker or £600 to the spirit drinker.) It is also argued that the optimal tax rate may well depend, for similar reasons, inversely on the income elasticity of demand[22]. Economic efficiency would, therefore, tend to indicate the taxing of commodities in inverse relation to their price and income elasticities of demand. For the UK, and probably for most economies, cigarettes and other tobacco products have both relatively low price and income elasticities of demand (the average for all goods and services being 1.0) and so, on grounds of economic efficiency alone, there is a strong case for shifting taxes from other commodities to tobacco. This does not include considerations of equity (which may indicate the opposite), nor of health (which would favour the shift).

Tax policies may or should also consider external costs or factors not taken into account by individuals in their consumption decisions, but borne by others in society. One criterion may be to set a tax such that consumers would choose the level of consumption they would have chosen, had they to pay the relevant (external) costs. These externalities include real resource costs, such as extra costs of health services (estimated at £610 million per annum in the UK)[23], costs of fires caused by tobacco smoking (£20 million per annum for the UK)[24] and loss of real output not borne by the smoker (50 million working days per annum in the UK)[24]. They may also be considered to include externalities of transfer payments such as retirement pensions, pensions to dependants and sickness and invalidity welfare payments (net £190 million per annum in the UK)[25]. They would not include tobacco tax as this is included in the price the smoker actually pays and is willing to pay for tobacco. These approximate estimates of externality costs of about £800 million per annum would support an **extra** tax for social costs or externalities in the region of £0.20 per packet in the UK.

Tobacco tax has fallen in importance in its contribution to UK Government revenue due to the increase in revenue from other sources and the fall in tobacco consumption for reasons other than tax rises, so that whereas in 1950 tobacco tax provided 16% of all Government revenue, this fell to 8% by the late 1960s, is currently 3.6% and may be even less significant by the end of the century.

Smoking, taxation and poverty

Before the widespread publicity about the health effects of smoking in the early 1960s, there was little difference between the smoking habits of different socioeconomic groups, but in the UK and in some other countries, smoking prevalence is now highest among people in poor socioeconomic circumstances. The decline in UK smoking rates over the last few decades has been relatively low among such people. Survey results suggest that smoking rates are particularly high among the unemployed[26] and young adults with families, especially lone parents[27]. Families with low incomes tend to have high smoking rates, and to spend a disproportionately large share of their income on cigarettes. Smoking, therefore, decreases the resources available to them more generally as well as directly harming their health.

The differential health effects are quite clear, particularly for mortality from smoking-induced disease. A man in an unskilled manual occupation in the UK is more than 4 times as likely to die of lung cancer as a professional, and twice as likely to die from coronary heart disease. For women there is a 3-fold difference for lung cancer and a 4-fold difference for heart disease[8]. For lung cancer, heart disease and chronic bronchitis, the inequalities between manual and non-manual groups widened between 1971 and 1981.

As we have seen, response to price tends to be particularly high among people in disadvantaged circumstances and, on average, they are likely to reduce not only levels of consumption but also total expenditure on cigarettes when there is a price rise. Raising relative prices would be expected to narrow the differentials in smoking prevalence and consumption between social and economic groups. Unfortunately, a direct consequence of such policies would be to further reduce the effective spending ability of people in poverty if they continue to smoke at the same rate.

This presents a dilemma. Should the price of cigarettes be held down to avoid hardship to families in poor economic circumstances? The difficulty with this is that price does have most effect on smoking by lower income groups, where health education has had the least. Erosion of cigarette prices could be seriously detrimental to public health, particularly to the health of lower income groups. The dynamic relationship between smoking, health and inequalities stretches over a lifetime and price is a potential force to break this link at any stage, reducing the harmful effects in terms of smokers' health and that of their children. A rational solution may be to increase benefits to poor families such as lone mothers, as well as raising cigarette prices. This would provide a disincentive to smoke without a detrimental effect on living standards. Expenditure on cigarettes would mostly be clawed back to the government through the tobacco tax. More work is necessary to find ways of ameliorating these problems.

Conclusion

There is little doubt that price has a major effect on cigarette consumption and thus smoking induced disease, especially in low income groups. To use this as a tool of preventive medicine, therefore, seems the right public health policy[28]. Fiscal policy is not an alternative to other methods of reducing the harm of tobacco, but it is one of the most powerful elements of the type of comprehensive policy recommended by the World Health Organization and other authoritative bodies. Raising tobacco tax also has the advantage to governments of increasing revenue. Public information and health promotion campaigns reduce smoking in their own right; they may also pave the way to make cigarette tax increases for health reasons politically acceptable. Progressive increases in taxes will reduce smoking and smoking disease, to the interest of health in all countries. Special measures may be necessary to ameliorate effects on the cost of living of poor families.

References

1   Central Statistical Office. *National Income and Expenditure Accounts*. London: HMSO, 1972–93

2   *INSEE Comptes Nationaux Dominique Darman*. Paris: INSEE Première No. 100 August 1990

3   Sweanor D. *Canadian Tobacco Tax Project*. Ottawa: Non-Smokers Rights Association, 1985–91

4   Saloojee Y. Price and income elasticity of demand for cigarettes in South Africa. In: Slama K. ed. *Tobacco and Health*. New York: Plenum, 1995: In press

5   Andrews RL, Franke GR. The determinants of cigarette consumption: a meta-analysis. *J Public Policy Marketing* 1991; 81–100

6   Lewit EM, Coate D. The potential for using excise taxes to reduce smoking. *J Health Economics* 1982; **1**: 121–45

7   Wasserman J, Manning WE, Newhouse JP, Winkler JD. The effects of excise taxes and regulation on cigarette smoking. *J Health Economics* 1991; **1**: 43–64

8   Townsend J, Roderick P, Cooper J. Cigarette smoking by socioeconomic group, sex and age: effects of price, income and health publicity. *BMJ* 1994; **309**: 923–27

9   Atkinson AB, Gomulka J, Stern N. *Household expenditure on tobacco 1970–1980: evidence from the family expenditure survey*. London: London School of Economics, 1984

10 Fry V, Pashardes P. *Changing patterns of smoking: are there economic causes?* London: Institute of Fiscal Studies, 1988

11 Secretary of State for Health. *The Health of the Nation: a Strategy for Health in England* (white paper). London: HMSO, 1992

12 Townsend J. Policies to halve smoking deaths. *Addiction* 1993; **88**: 43–52

13 Bolling K. *Smoking among Secondary School Children in England in 1993*. London: HMSO, 1994

14 European Bureau for Action on Smoking Prevention (BASP). Newsletter 24. Brussels: BASP, 1994: pp 7–8

15 Townsend J. *Price, Tax and Smoking in Europe*. Copenhagen: World Health Organization, 1988

16 Townsend J. Cigarette taxation and single European market. *BMJ* 1992; **307**: 587.

17 Joosens L, Raw M. Smuggling and cross border shopping of tobacco in Europe. *BMJ* 1995; **310**: 1393–7

18 Jones A, Posnet J. The revenue and welfare effects of cigarette taxes. *Appl Economics* 1988; 1223–32

19 Ramsey FA. A mathematical theory of savings. *Economic J* 1928; 38

20 Baumal WJ, Bradford DF. Optimal departures from marginal cost pricing. *Am Economic Rev* 1970: 60

21 Kay JA, King MA. *The British Tax System*. 5th edn. Oxford: Open University Press, 1990

22 Atkinson AB, Stiglitz JE. *Lectures on Public Economics*. London: McGraw Hill, 1980

23 Health Education Authority. *The Smoking Epidemic*. London: Health Education Authority, 1993

24 ASH Fact Sheet No 3. *Economics of Smoking*. 1995

25 Townsend J. Social cost, externalities and tobacco taxation in UK. *CDC Economist meeting on Optimal Taxation*. Boston: 1995

26 Office of Population Censuses and Surveys. *General Household Survey*. London: HMSO, 1972 to 1994

27 Marsh A, McKay S. *Poor Smokers*. London: Institute of Policy Studies, 1994

28 Townsend J. The burden of smoking. In: Benzeval M, Judge K, Whitehead M, eds. *Tackling Inequalities in Health*. London: King's Fund Institute, 1995: pp 82–94

Tobacco and the law: the state of the art

Gillian Howard

Consultant, Mishcon De Reya, Solicitors, London, UK

Litigation has become a major weapon in the conflict between those who seek to control tobacco and the tobacco industry. Apart from the cases arising from the high proportion of fires caused by cigarettes (including, in the UK, the disastrous fire at the Bradford football stadium and the fire at Kings Cross railway station, both of which were caused by discarded cigarette butts), in the last few years there have been and are continuing major lawsuits against the tobacco manufacturers both in the USA and in the UK. In Australia, a Court has ruled that the tobacco industry's claims that passive smoke had not been proven to cause a variety of diseases were false and misleading. A Quebec judge ruled as unconstitutional a Canadian law which had banned tobacco advertising. A product liability suit was filed against cigarette manufacturers by airline flight attendants whose health, they alleged, was impaired by exposure to passive smoke.

To date, attempts to win damages from the manufacturers for injuries caused by smoking have failed, but several group actions are pending in the courts in England and the USA. The cases to date demonstrate the range and importance of tobacco control issues now being considered by the Courts.

Historical perspective

Any controls in the UK over the use of tobacco in the workplace and in public places have largely been voluntary. As far back as 8 March 1824, Lord Palmerston ordered that no person should smoke in the office during office hours[1]. It is also well recorded that King James I detested and discouraged smoking at Court.

The only positive 'right' to smoke expressly set out in English law is to be found in the Execution of Sentences (Army, Navy and Airforce) Regulations 1956[2] which give a traitor condemned to death the right to the last rites, a visit from his family and a last cigarette!

Recently, several major airlines including British Airways have banned smoking on internal flights and several US airlines have extended the ban on internal flights to transatlantic flights as well. In the UK, recent Regulations have banned smoking on buses and trams[3]. But whilst several attempts have been made to pass legislation banning smoking in workplaces and public places, these have so far failed[4].

'Innocent victims' of smoking

Apart from the active smoker, who until 1971 had never been warned by the tobacco companies about the dangers of tobacco products, there are two classes of innocent victims of smoking — the unborn child of a mother who smokes (these babies are likely to have low-birth weight with associated susceptibilities to illness) and the passive smoker. This second category of victim is now known to be at a substantial risk of the same range of tobacco-induced illnesses as an active smoker[5].

Government controls

In the UK, there are limited Governmental controls over tobacco products based in the main on voluntary agreements between Government and the tobacco industry. In 1971, the tobacco industry moved to head off possible legislation and litigation by agreeing with the Department of Health and Social Security (DHSS) to print on cigarette packets: 'WARNING BY HM GOVERNMENT. SMOKING CAN DAMAGE YOUR HEALTH'. On all cigarette advertisements, there is a statement: 'every packet carries a Government health warning'.

This has been renegotiated several times since, but its essence remains the same. More recently, the original warning has had 'cigarettes' substituted for 'smoking' and has been stiffened by the adverb 'seriously'. Warnings such as 'most doctors don't smoke' have been added. In addition, warnings are also given as to the risk of harm to the fetus during pregnancy. Health warnings on cigarette packets are now governed by Regulations[6]. In a European Court of Justice (ECJ) case in 1993, several tobacco manufacturers sought to have ruled void the UK Regulations relating to warning notices which require larger notices than specified in the European Directive. The challenge was unsuccessful. The ECJ held that Member States are at liberty to decide that the Government health warning ought to be larger than that required by European Directive 'in view of the level of public awareness of the health issues associated with tobacco consumption'[7].

However, the European Union's Resolution seeking that Member States ban smoking in public places has not been adopted by the UK and is unlikely to be so[9].

Ironically, the statutory controls over who is permitted to buy tobacco products means that the most serious penalty is for those who sell tobacco products to children aged less than 16 years!

Personal injury claims – the active smoker

An active smoker with small cell lung cancer would be a prime candidate to bring a claim for negligence against the tobacco manufacturer(s), based in the law of tort. A tort is an actionable wrong at common law. The wrongdoer does something which is foreseeably going to cause harm to someone else, to whom the wrongdoer owes a duty of care and for which it was reasonable in the circumstances to take steps to avoid doing it[9].

'State of the art'

The Courts judge the question of negligence on the state of the knowledge at the time when it is alleged the harm was caused (or commenced). In 1950, the work of Sir Richard Doll and Austin Bradford Hill revealed that there was a causal link between smoking and lung cancer and, in 1957, after much further work had been reported, the Medical Research Council advised the government that cigarette smoking was the cause of the increased mortality from lung cancer. In 1962, the Royal College of Physicians reviewed the evidence for a harmful effect of smoking and concluded that the total death rate was greatly increased in smokers and that there was a causal link not only with lung cancer, but also with bronchitis, heart disease and tuberculosis. In 1964, the US Surgeon General published a report which came to the same conclusions. In 1988, Sir Peter Froggatt published the Report of the Independent Scientific Committee into the health effects for passive smokers.

What are the acts of negligence?

It is arguable that the tobacco manufacturers committed several acts and omissions which amount to negligence:

- firstly, by not warning their consumers of the risks until 1971, when the state of the art was established back in 1957, so that the consumers could exercise consumer choice.

- secondly, by continuing to manufacture and market high-tar cigarettes and failing to minimise their harm irrespective of consumer choice.
- thirdly, by continuing to manufacture and market cigarettes.

If the claim for negligence was limited to failure to warn, then liability expires or shrinks at 1971 when warnings were printed on cigarette boxes. Here claims for negligence may be defeated if the defendant can show that, even if the appropriate precautions had been taken by the defendant, the plaintiff would have ignored or failed to use them — Cummings vs Sir William Arrol[10]. It may be arguable on behalf of a smoker that (s)he had become addicted in the mid 1950s, had made several unsuccessful attempts to give up and, therefore, it would be established that printed warnings would have been of no use.

The failure to reduce the tar level in cigarettes would only be a relevant matter if the plaintiff continued to smoke only high-tar cigarettes.

The third possible claim, that it was negligent to continue to manufacture and market cigarettes, is fraught with difficulties. Whilst there is nothing in principle to stop a Court finding that a product is so dangerous that it is negligent to make or market it, it is unrealistic to expect the judicial process to shut down the whole of the tobacco industry. What the Courts may require are better safeguards and at an earlier stage than were actually taken.

How do negligence claims succeed?

For a claim in negligence to succeed, the plaintiff must show a duty of care is owed to them, that duty of care has been breached and the harm that they have suffered has been caused by that breach of the duty of care[11]. The burden of proof is on the balance of probabilities. Is it more likely that an active smoker's lung cancer was caused by the tobacco products or not?

In assessing the knowledge that a defendant ought to possess, the Courts have made it clear that even the remotest risk, once it is or should have been appreciated, puts a duty on anyone responsible for it to take whatever preventive measures were practicable and proportionate to the risk. The Privy Council made this principle clear in The Wagon Mound No 2[12].

Any smoker who seeks legal redress for harm caused prior to 1957 is unlikely to succeed. However, those who continued to buy cigarettes after 1957, the point in time when there was established knowledge of risk, and in 1971 when manufacturers began to publish health warnings, must have a strong case for establishing that the manufacturers knew of the risks of lung cancer from 1957 and at the very least ought to have warned their consumers of those risks[13].

In a landmark ruling in the US, the Supreme Court ruled that the health warnings on cigarette packets do not automatically protect the manufacturers from being sued by the victims of smoking[14].

It may well be arguable that the tobacco manufacturers were negligent in continuing to manufacture unnecessarily dangerous high-tar cigarettes after 1957, particularly in light of the fact that in those days the manufacturers did not publish the tar levels. It may be argued that liability in this respect may go back as far as 1955, when experimental evidence was published indicating that the principal carcinogenic components of tobacco smoke were found in the tarry fraction.

For a plaintiff with lung cancer who has smoked 40 cigarettes a day for decades, even the most bullish of medical experts used by defendants to contest lung disease cases is likely to admit defeat in the light of the present statistical knowledge and of the recent 'all or nothing decision in the House of Lords in Hotson vs East Berkshire Health Authority[15].

In this case, it was established that if a plaintiff would have suffered lasting injury in any event, a negligent act which ensures that he does so, is not on balance of probability, responsible for his final condition. As a necessary corollary it must be arguable that where more probably than not the plaintiff would be in good health but for the defendant's acts or omissions, the defendant is liable if his acts or omissions were negligent.

But, beyond this, there is a now a soundly established body of law which relieves a plaintiff of the need to pin either the entire blame or a proportion of it on the defendant — McGhee vs National Coal Board[16].

Both the Hotson and McGhee cases establish that the defendants are not entitled to any discount for the extent to which they did not contribute to the risk. This means that the defendant gains nothing by pointing to other contributory or alternative causes of lung disease unless the evidence is strong enough to make the proof of them disproof of the materiality of smoking to the plaintiff's condition. In other words, the plaintiff need go no further than proving that more probably than not the smoking of the defendant's cigarettes has materially contributed to his ill-health.

Two caveats

The Courts will attribute the damage to health to two distinct periods, the pre-negligent and negligent period[17]. In other words, the tobacco manufacturers may seek to argue that the latent damage was all done prior to 1957, in the early years of the smoker's life and so the manufacturers should carry no liability.

The tobacco manufacturers may also argue for an apportionment of damages to exclude the damage done in the pre-negligent period. Even if both these arguments succeed, they will not defeat a claim but only diminish the damages awarded.

Hoist with their own petard

The defendants in any litigation are bound to attack the research before 1971 (as they continue to do in 1995), taking their classic stance that the findings of the research before this date were ambivalent, it would have been wrong to alarm the consumer and their mutually exclusive duties to their shareholders and employees.

However, they may be hoist with their own petard. Their success in dissuading the Government from imposing statutory controls on tar levels or statutory requirements of printed warnings means that they have no benchmark of implied statutory licence.

In a case involving Shell and BP, Budden vs BP and Shell[18], the Court accepted the defendants' argument that they could not be held to be negligent for the damage caused to two children alleged to come from the lead content of petrol fumes because the lead content of their petrol fell within the prescribed limits set out by regulations having the force of law[19]. They were in effect immunised against negligence claims even if the lead content could be proved to do foreseeable harm. The fact that warnings have, since 1966, been required under the Federal Cigarette Labelling and Advertising Act in the US has likewise saved the manufacturers there from claims for failing to warn.

Exemplary damages

Damages awarded for the harm caused by tobacco products could be significant. For pain and suffering, the Courts would take into account the agony of contemplating an early death. They will also reflect the loss of earnings and of future earnings for a living plaintiff and his/her dependants.

One of the few classes of case in which exemplary damages are available to punish or make an example of a wrongdoer is the case of defendant who has knowingly committed a tort in the expectation that the profits to be made outweigh the risk of being sued or stopped — Rookes vs Barnard[20].

UK group action

A group presently comprising some 200 English smokers believe that their various illnesses are caused by smoking and are commencing a claim for negligence against several English tobacco companies[21]. Their claim is that the manufacturers failed to take any or any sufficient steps to reduce the risks, nor did they give adequate warnings of them. The plaintiffs say that, from the 1950s at least, the tobacco industry knew or ought to have known that smoking caused many diseases and that the warnings from 1971 initially misled the public about its risks, merely saying that 'smoking can damage your health'.

Legal aid of £100,000 has now been granted in respect of 200 smokers so that, in the first instance, expert opinion may be sought on the effect of advertising and warnings and other matters connected with failure to reduce the nicotine content of cigarettes. Leading defence counsel have pointed out that there are several hurdles to surmount. The smokers will have to show that he or she did not know of the dangers of smoking; that they tried to give up; that their injury was caused by smoking; and that their claim is not out of time because it was launched more than 3 years after the plaintiff first knew of the injury.

Litigation in US: class actions

Recent litigation in the US is based upon the addictive effects of nicotine. Cases are now being brought against manufacturers for their failure to warn of the risks of smoking including the risk of addiction, and/or for the failure to take steps to reduce the risks. In the US, class actions are likely to increase the power of litigants by combining resources and expertise.

In February 1995, the New Orleans Court permitted a class action to be brought in the name of Castano against an American tobacco company on behalf of over 100 million smokers, including those living and the estates of persons who have died from smoking related illness. The case is brought on behalf of the plaintiff and 'all other nicotine-dependent persons' seeking punitive damages as well as compensation for economic loss, emotional distress and medical costs arising out of the fact that tobacco companies (including Philip Morris, RJ Reynolds and a subsidiary of BAT) had concealed their knowledge of the addictive capacity of nicotine. It is estimated that damages could run to $50 billion[22].

Passive smoking

The harm

The significant harm caused by passive smoking has been further established, following the Froggatt Report, in a US study into environmental tobacco smoke published by the Environmental Protection Agency[23]. The Report states that about 3000 US non smokers die every year from lung cancer caused by exposure to tobacco fumes. In addition, between 150,000–300,000 cases of bronchitis and pneumonia in children under 18 months of age are reported each year.

Also in the US, the Florida Appeal Court has ruled that a class action may proceed by 30 non-smoking airline cabin crew, representative of 600,000 fellow employees, against various tobacco companies[24]. The plaintiffs state that they were obliged to inhale environment tobacco smoke on flights where smoking was permitted. They now suffer from diseases attributed to passive smoking, including lung cancer, asthma and other diseases. Damages are sought in the region of $5 billion. The case is of interest as it is the first time that the American courts have recognised possible harm from passive smoking.

Claims against employers

Probably one of the best-known claims for passive smoking against an employer involved Mr Sean Carroll, an Australian bus driver, who sued his employers on account of his lung cancer caused, he claimed, by 35 years' exposure to the tobacco fumes of his passengers and co-workers. He accepted an out-of-court settlement of $65,000 and died one year after the settlement[25].

In another well-publicized case involving a British woman, Veronica Bland, Stockport Metropolitan Borough Council made an out-of-court settlement of £15,000 to her after proceedings had been issued for negligence and breach of statutory duty. She alleged that she had suffered serious health complaints, including chronic bronchitis, which she alleged was caused by her exposure to passive smoke[26].

More recently, Chartered West LB Ltd, an investment bank in the City of London made an out of court settlement of £2,500 to one of its employees who had a long history of asthma. The Employment Department had recommended that as registered disabled, she should work in a smoke-free environment. However, other employees smoked around her and she eventually was forced into hospital with severe asthma[27].

In an Australian case, Scholem vs New South Wales Health Department[28], a Court awarded $85,000 to a plaintiff who had alleged that her employers had negligently caused her to contract lung disease by requiring her to work with colleagues who smoked.

And . . . , an irate non-smoker who was made uncomfortable by cigarette smoke from the room adjacent to that in which his daughter was recovering from an operation was awarded damages of £50 against the private hospital which permitted smoking in patients' rooms[29].

It is not, perhaps, surprising that following the publicity about these cases, many more employers in the UK have introduced bans or radical restrictions on smoking in their workplaces.

Other legal actions for smokers

Smokers may consider bringing a legal action under the *Sale of Goods Act 1979* or the *Consumer Protection Act 1987*. Under the Sale of Goods Act, it is an offence not to sell goods of a merchantable quality and defects must specifically be drawn to the buyer's attention before the contract is made[30]. The goods must also be fit for the purpose for which they are bought. It is arguable that under the Limitation Act 1980 s.11, it is possible for a smoker to sue on a contract for the sale of cigarettes made before the health warnings were published by the manufacturers, provided that the injury to health has only recently manifested itself.

It may be that since warnings have been placed on cigarette packets since 1971, it is only pre-1971 contracts of sale which are actionable. It may be that any action has more likelihood of success for negligence.

The Consumer Protection Act 1987 introduced product liability, making the producer of a product liable for any damage caused wholly or partly by a defect in the goods. However, s.10(7) excludes various potentially or actually dangerous products including medicinal products and tobacco — the industry has evidently succeeded in nipping this form of liability in the bud!

Employer's duties to the workforce

The criminal law

There is no positive legal protection for workers to work in a smoke-free environment, neither is there an overall legal duty on employers to ban or restrict smoking in the workplace. There are some specific prohibitions on smoking at workplaces where, for example, flammable materials, gas, radioactive materials and chemicals[31] are present.

The Health and Safety at Work Act 1974 requires employers to provide a safe place of work, a safe system of work and a safe working environment so far as is reasonably practicable[32]. Health and Safety Regulations which came into force on 1 January 1993, derived from European Directives, hardly mention smoking as a health issue save for one reference where smoking is described as a 'discomfort'. Here, employers must provide a separate rest rooms and rest areas for non-smokers in order to 'protect non-smokers from discomfort caused by tobacco smoke'[33]. It is a curious anomaly that this still leaves the areas dedicated to work not being subjected to any express statutory control on smoking.

Under the Management of Health and Safety at Work Regulations[34], there is a duty upon employers to carry out risk assessments on 'significant and substantial risks' and adopt control measures to eliminate or reduce the risk. It is highly arguable, that the risk of exacerbating asthma for those who already suffer and the increased risk of lung cancer for non-smokers is a significant risk. Whether the Health and Safety Executive (HSE) would take action against employers who had failed to address the risk of passive smoking under these Regulations is debatable. The view of the HSE appears to be that whilst 'Health and Safety Inspectors can take enforcement action if necessary in these circumstances, ultimately it would be for the courts to decide in a particular case whether the risk to health was significant'.

The Courts view what is reasonably practicable in terms of the quantum of risk, in this case, the risk to non-smokers of contracting lung cancer, exacerbating or causing asthma and other chest complaints, causing or making worse eye complaints, etc., with the time, trouble and expense in averting that risk. It could be argued that it is cost effective and cost-saving for any employer to ban or restrict smoking in his office, factory or workshops since this would reduce the risk of accidental fire, reduce the cleaning costs and would reduce absenteeism amongst both smokers and passive smokers. This argument has yet to be tested.

This Health and Safety at Work Act imposes criminal sanctions — fines and imprisonment — on employers and also upon directors and managers if they consent or connive in any breach of their statutory duty, and also upon workers. Workers must take reasonable care of their own and others' health and safety and co-operate with their employer over matters of health and safety and not to intentionally or recklessly interfere with anything provided in the interests of health and safety (ss.7 and 8).

In addition to fines and terms of imprisonment for breaching the statutory duties, the Health and Safety Inspectors and Environment Health Officers who enforce the Act in respect of factories and offices respectively have the power to issue Improvement and Prohibition Notices on workplaces and on individuals. There have been rare cases where the threat of such Notices has prompted employers to introduce no smoking policies[35]. There have to date been no prosecutions under this Act for permitting smoking in the workplace.

The Health and Safety Executive (HSE) has published a second edition of its booklet *Passive Smoking at Work* relying mainly on the voluntary action of employers to introduce no smoking policies rather than threaten legal action under the Health and Safety at Work Act.

Smoking and recruitment

Since the law in the UK at present only recognises limited forms of discrimination as unlawful, for example on the grounds of sex (*Sex Discrimination Act 1974*) or race (*Race Relations Act 1975*) and discrimination for permanent disability (*Disability Discrimination Act 1995*), it is not unlawful for employers to seek to recruit only non-smokers or to discriminate against smokers who might wish to smoke at work. This could be one way for employers to introduce a policy of non-smoking.

Introducing no smoking policies

Employers are required to act carefully when proposing new rules which would either ban or restrict smoking in the workplace. They must take care not to breach their workers' contracts of employment and not to offend the employment protection legislation which protects employees from unfair dismissal if they are dismissed for refusing to comply with any new no smoking rules.

Where an employer chooses to impose a smoking ban in the workplace, employees who are dedicated smokers have sometimes found that they are unable to cope with the new conditions, leave their jobs and claim constructive dismissal, alleging that the employer has unilaterally changed a fundamental term of the contract of employment making it impossible for them to continue working.

In Dryden vs Greater Glasgow Health Board[36], (the only appellate decision on this point) the employee, a nurse, who was prevented from smoking at work when a no smoking policy was introduced, was held not to have been constructively dismissed. The Employment Appeal Tribunal held there is no implied term in a contract of employment permitting an employee to smoke at work.

> The introduction of a no smoking policy did not constitute a breach of . . . contract. . . . There was no specific implied term . . . that she would be entitled to have access to facilities for smoking during working hours. . . . The rule against smoking was lawful. . . . The fact that it bears hardly on a particular employee does not . . . justify an inference that the employer has acted in such a way as to repudiate the contract . . .

Action by the State

In countries other than UK, the State has taken action to restrict smoking in public places. The criminal law has been invoked in Western Australia by the Department of Occupational Health, Safety and Welfare under state legislation following complaints by employees of a gambling casino that they were subjected to passive smoke. The maximum penalty under statute is $50,000.

In France, legislation passed in 1992 places severe restrictions upon smoking in public places including trains, planes and restaurants.

In Norway, additional legislation was passed in 1987 tightening up the Norwegian Tobacco Act of 1973 imposing a ban on smoking in all public places.

In the USA, the states of Mississippi, Minnesota, Florida and West Virginia are suing the American tobacco companies, claiming punitive damages, reimbursement of past health care of victims of smoking related disease, compensation for future cost of health care for current and future victims and injunctions forbidding the promotion of cigarettes to minors.

The aim is to recover the enormous and increasing outlay of individual states on treating tobacco-related disease. West Virginia's health budget for smoking related illness is presently $500 million per year, and Minnesota spends $350 million. Minnesota and the Blue Cross Health Insurance Company are jointly suing to recover welfare and health insurance expenditure arising from smoking-related illnesses, alleging that the tobacco industry illegally hid the health hazards of cigarettes and manipulated nicotine levels to ensure that customers would become addicted. Similar cases are being brought by Mississippi and Florida.

Other claims

In New South Wales, Australia, Dr Sarah Hodson is claiming A$1,000 from WD & HO Wills for treatment for nicotine addiction. However, the tobacco company is disputing the claim and has succeeded in their application for the matter to be heard in a higher court. The hearing will take place in late 1995, if Dr Hodson has the resources to pay for the increased level of costs of continuing her case in the higher court.

Deskiewickz vs Philip Morris is a similar current case in the US, in which the plaintiff is suing for $1,153 to cover the cost of medical treatment for nicotine patches and health club membership fees. He claims that Philip Morris owed him a duty of care to warn him that nicotine is addictive and that he would require treatment to enable him to stop smoking.

Conclusion

The tobacco manufacturers will fight the cases against them with vigour, as success for any plaintiff, whether on the small or large scale of damages, will open the flood-gates of litigation.

With the onus of proving that smoking was not the main cause of a plaintiff's illness, defence experts will become increasingly hard put to justify the use of tobacco products, especially if the US Food and Drug Administration declares that nicotine is a drug whose levels should be reduced to non-addictive levels, probably zero. They will need to be aware of the Finnish doctor who gave evidence to support the defendants in a smoking case and is now being charged with perjury[37].

Acknowledgements

With thanks to Linda Goldman LLB, Barrister at Law, 7 Stone Buildings, Lincoln's Inn, London WC2A 3SZ, UK, for additional research and most valuable assistance.

References

1   Foreign Office, 8 March 1824; from the Chief Clerk: 'I have been directed by Lord Palmerston to desire that a peremptory stop may from this time forward be put to all smoking in the office during office hours. Be so good as to convey this Order to the Heads of Departments and to desire that they will stop the practise of smoking in their several Departments; and that they will export any person who shall hereafterward contravene Lord Palmerston's order'

2   *Execution of Sentences of Death (Army) Regulations 1956* SI 1956 No.1970, Regulation 8 (h), *Execution of Sentences of Death (Airforce) Regulations 1956* SI 1956 No. 2054, Regulation 8 (h), *Execution of Sentences of Death (Navy) Regulations 1956* SI 1956 No. 62

3   *The Public Service Vehicles (Conduct of Drivers, Inspectors, Conductors and Passengers) Regulations 1990* SI 1990 No. 1020, Regulation 6 (d)

4   Mr George Foulkes, Labour MP for Cumnock and Doon Valley, sponsored a Private Member's Bill seeking to control smoking at work in the Health and Safety at Work (Tobacco Smoking) Bill, on 2 March 1992

5   Fourth Report of the Independent Scientific Committee – Smoking and Health (Chairman, Sir Peter Froggatt). London: HMSO, 1988

6   *Tobacco Products Labelling (Safety) Regulations 1991* SI 1991 No. 1530, Regulation 5(2)(d)

7   R vs Secretary of State for Health ex parte Gallaher Ltd and others. *ECJ, The Times* 28 June 1993

8   EC Mixed Resolution on *Banning Smoking in Places open to the Public* (89/C/189/01)

9   Winfield and Jolowicz on Tort, 12th edn. p 69

10 Cummings vs Sir William Arrol. *Weekly Law Report* 1962; **1**: 295

11 The 'neighbour' principle as expounded by Lord Atkin in Donoghue vs Stevenson. *Appeal Cases* 1932 562; Peabody Fund Governors vs Sir Lindsay Parkinson. *Appeal Cases* 1985; 240: 'in determining whether or not a duty of care of particular scope was incumbent upon a defendant it is material to take into consideration whether it is just and reasonable that it should be so'

12 The Wagon Mound. *Appeal Cases* 1967; **2**: 617

13 Thompson vs Smiths Shiprepairers. *Queens Bench* 1984; 405: Wilsher vs Essex Area Health Authority. *Weekly Law Report* 1987; **2**: 425

14 *The Times* 25 June 1992

15 Hotson vs East Berkshire Health Authority. *Weekly Law Report* 1987; **3**: 232

16 McGhee vs National Coal Board. *Weekly Law Report* 1973; **1**: 1

17 Thompson's case (see above)

18 Budden vs BP and Shell. *Solicitors Law J* 1980; **124**: 376
19 *Control of Pollution Act 1974*
20 Rookes vs Barnard. *Appeal Case* 1964; 1029
21 *The Times* 30 June 1992
22 *Financial Times* 18 February 1995
23 *Financial Times* 8 November 1993
24 *Guardian* 14 December 1994
25 Sean Carroll vs Melbourne Transit Authority. Public statement made by Mr Bernard Murphy, Solicitor of Slater & Gordon, 11 August 1988
26 Veronica Bland vs Stockport Metropolitan Borough Council. Settled January 1993
27 *The Times* 4 August 1994
28 *Sydney Morning Herald* 28 May 1992
29 Terry Hurlstone. *The Times* 11 April 1994
30 *Sales of Goods Act 1979*; s.14(2); s.14(6). *Sale of Goods (Implied Terms) Act 1973*, s.7(2)
31 Examples of such Regulations are: *Highly Flammable Liquids and Liquefied Petroleum Gases Regulations 1972; Ionising Radiation Regulations 1985* and *Gas Safety (Installation and Use) Regulations 1994*
32 *The Health and Safety at Work Act 1974*, s.2(1)
33 *Workplace, Health, Safety and Welfare Regulations 1992*, Regulation 25 (3)
34 *Management of Health and Safety at Work Regulations 1992*, Regulation 3
35 Paul Hooper, Environmental Health Officer working for Birmingham City Council, reported in the *Independent* 23 March 1988
36 Dryden vs Greater Glasgow Health Board. *Industrial Relations Law Reports* 1992; **469**
37 Aurejarvi E. *The Battle in Finland Against the Tobacco Industry.* Paris: 9th World Conference 1994

Strategies for smoking cessation

Jonathan Foulds

Division of Addictive Behaviour, St George's Hospital Medical School, London, UK

Smoking cessation strategies should be geared to the target group's level of motivation to quit, and degree of tobacco addiction. Motivational interventions (e.g. media campaigns) aim to encourage more people to try to stop smoking. Treatment interventions (e.g. nicotine replacement) aim to increase the chances of a quit attempt being successful. In populations which have already been saturated by motivational interventions, the overall effect of adding further motivational interventions may be rather small, and possibly non-existent in heavy smokers. As a population's smoking prevalence declines, so the balance of interventions should shift from motivational to treatment approaches. Nicotine replacement is an effective smoking cessation aid and should form the basis for treating moderate to heavy smokers. There may be a case for the development of more specialist clinics to treat motivated but addicted smokers and train health professionals how to apply effective smoking cessation methods as part of their routine work.

The four main methods of reducing the health consequences of tobacco are: (i) reducing the number of people who initiate tobacco use; (ii) increasing the number of tobacco users who stop; (iii) increasing the number of continuing tobacco users who switch to less harmful forms of tobacco use; and (iv) decreasing non-smokers' exposure to environmental tobacco smoke. This paper will focus on describing and evaluating interventions designed to promote smoking cessation, which can potentially be carried out by health professionals.

Smokers generally do not stop smoking without first deciding that this is a desirable outcome and making a conscious decision to do so. However, it has become clear that a large proportion of smokers who decide that they would like to stop smoking and make attempts to do so are unsuccessful. Before going on to describe and evaluate the various types of smoking cessation interventions which exist, it is appropriate to consider in some detail two of the main factors which determine whether or not an individual smoker stops smoking: **motivation** (desire/intention to stop smoking) and **addiction** (compulsive smoking characterised by impaired voluntary control, also often called 'dependence').

Motivation

A smoker's motivation (drive, intention, desire) to stop smoking is clearly a critical factor in whether or not they are likely to quit. There are two commonly used methods of assessing this factor. The first method consists of asking smokers a few simple questions about the strength of their desire to stop smoking. Two typical multiple choice questions[1] are given below, along with a suggested scoring format:

(a) *Would you give up smoking altogether, if you could do so easily?*

Yes, definitely	Yes, probably	Possibly	Probably not	Definitely not
(4)	(3)	(2)	(1)	(0)

(b) *How much do you want to stop smoking altogether?*

Not at all	Slightly	Moderately	Quite strongly	Very strongly
(0)	(1)	(2)	(3)	(4)

A number of studies[1,2] have found (not surprisingly) that likelihood of successful cessation is predicted by total motivation scores like those given above.

The other method of assessing motivation to change is that implicit in the 'Stage of Change' model of human behaviour[3]. This model recognises that, like many other behaviours, smoking cessation is often better described as a cyclical activity than as a discrete event. It is suggested that smokers typically progress through five stages described below: **Precontemplation**: currently smoking and not seriously considering quitting within the next six months. **Contemplation**: currently smoking and seriously considering quitting within the next six months (but not within the next thirty days). **Preparation**: Currently smoking and seriously intending to quit within the next thirty days. **Action**: Not currently smoking, having quit in the last six months. **Maintenance**: Not currently smoking, having abstained for over six months.

Of course relapse is very common in smokers attempting to quit, causing them to re-enter the cycle again at some earlier stage. Again, this method of assessing motivation predicts likelihood of making an attempt to quit and likelihood of success in smokers exposed to a brief smoking cessation intervention[3].

There are some obvious merits to assessing the level of motivation/stage of change of the group of smokers to whom an intervention is being targeted. For example, it is clear that targeting an intensive smoking cessation treatment at smokers with no intention of quitting is likely to be a waste of time. It has been suggested that a better approach is to assess motivation and target appropriate interventions according to the target group/individual's level of motivation. For example, precontemplators

Table 1 DSMIV diagnostic criteria for nicotine withdrawal[8].

A. Daily use of nicotine for at least several weeks.
B. Abrupt cessation of nicotine use, or reduction in the amount of nicotine used, followed within 24 h by 4 (or more) of the following:
    (1) dysphoric or depressed mood
    (2) insomnia
    (3) irritability, frustration or anger
    (4) anxiety
    (5) difficulty concentrating
    (6) restlessness
    (7) decreased heart rate
    (8) increased appetite or weight gain
C. The symptoms in Criterion B cause clinically significant distress or impairment in social, occupational, or other important areas of functioning.
D. The symptoms are not due to a general medical condition and are not better accounted or by another mental disorder.

Associated features: craving for nicotine, desire for sweets, impaired performance on tasks requiring vigilance, EEG slowing, decrease in catecholamine and cortisol levels, decreased metabolism of some medications and other substances.

might be exposed to information on the health effects of tobacco together with the financial advantages of quitting, contemplators might be provided with information designed to tip their decisional balance in favour of quitting, along with materials giving advice on how to stop smoking, and people in the action stage might be given relapse prevention material. While this approach has considerable face validity, it has yet to be demonstrated to improve long term abstinence rates[4].

Addiction

Central to most definitions of drug addiction is the idea that it involves an element of compulsion (often in the face of serious adverse health consequences) and that it involves an impairment of self-control over the use of the drug (evidenced by failure to abstain despite high motivation and serious attempts to do so).

There is now a consensus amongst the medical and scientific communities that tobacco is addicting, that nicotine is the drug causing tobacco addiction, and that the mechanisms causing tobacco addiction are similar to those causing addiction to heroin and cocaine[5]. The evidence supporting this view is reviewed comprehensively in the 1988 US Surgeon General's Report, entitled *Nicotine Addiction*, but it is perhaps worth mentioning some of that evidence. The 1-year continuous abstinence rate for smokers making an unaided quit attempt is less than 5% [6,7]. It is therefore clear that most smokers find it difficult to stop smoking, even after they have made a conscious decision to do so.

When smokers abstain they frequently experience an unpleasant withdrawal syndrome, the main diagnostic features of which are shown in the Table. At least 49% of self-quitters and 68% of patients (smokers of at least 10 cigarettes per day) attempting to stop smoking with the help of their family doctor experience withdrawal symptoms meeting diagnostic criteria[8] for the nicotine withdrawal syndrome[9,10]. This withdrawal syndrome is relieved by nicotine administration (e.g. in the form of gum, nasal spray or skin patch) compared with placebo[10]. The proven efficacy of nicotine replacement as a smoking cessation aid (discussed below) is further evidence that many smokers are addicted to nicotine.

Like other addictions, tobacco addiction has degrees of severity which can be measured in a number of ways. Biochemical measures of nicotine consumption (e.g. blood nicotine or saliva cotinine concentration) sometimes provide the most powerful predictor of likelihood of success in any given quit attempt, but again a few brief questions about the time before smoking the first cigarette of the day, and daily cigarette consumption also provide good measures of tobacco dependence, which predict the difficulty an individual will have in stopping smoking[11,12]. If a smoker typically smokes at least 15 cigarettes per day or smokes their first cigarette of the day within half an hour of waking, then it is highly likely that they will find it difficult to stop smoking and will experience nicotine withdrawal symptoms on trying to do so.

When discussing smoking cessation interventions, it is important to consider which type of smoker the intervention is best targeted at, in terms of level of motivation to stop and degree of addiction to tobacco. In particular, it is important not to fall into the trap of comparing 'success rates' across interventions targeted at totally different groups of smokers.

Population based smoking cessation interventions

Community or population based smoking cessation projects generally aim to increase the number of smokers within the community who make an attempt to stop smoking, producing a net reduction in smoking prevalence within the target community. One assumption common to most community based interventions is that the important circumstances supporting a person's decision to smoke are social. Such interventions aim to create a social climate that does not support tobacco use, by intervening through social structures within a community. The intervention methods typically involve political, business and health leaders in the planning strategy, use of mass media to promote public education and campaign awareness, encouragement of health professionals to raise smoking as an issue with their patients, initiation of smoking cessation events (e.g. 'Quit and Win' contests) and provision of self-help materials (e.g. booklets and telephone quitlines) for smokers. Such interventions can be seen as trying to move the whole smoking population along the 'stage of change continuum' in the direction from 'precontemplation' towards maintained abstinence.

Such interventions have the advantage of being able to reach a sizeable proportion of the population. Even if only a small fraction of the smokers stop smoking as a result, this may still amount to a relatively large number, and hence a sizeable health gain.

Some studies of this type of intervention[13,14] have produced modest but encouraging results while others suggested that increased community education may be unlikely to improve upon secular reductions in smoking prevalence[15]. However, in order to illustrate some of the main issues involved in such interventions, particular attention will be paid here to the Community Intervention Trial for Smoking Cessation (COMMIT)[16,17]. At the time of writing this is the only such trial which focused on changing smoking behaviour (rather than a range of risk factors) and which involved random assignment within a sufficient number of community pairs to provide adequate statistical power to detect changes in smoking cessation rates using the community as the unit of analysis. It is probably the most extensive tobacco-control study yet undertaken.

The Community Intervention Trial for Smoking Cessation (COMMIT)

The COMMIT study took place in North America from 1989 to 1992. It aimed to evaluate whether a 4-year community-level intervention would increase quit-rates among cigarette smokers, with heavy smokers (>24 cigarettes per day) being a particular priority group. Twenty-two communities (populations in each ranged from 50,000 to 250,000) participated, forming eleven matched pairs. One of each pair was randomly assigned to receive the community intervention, while the other acted as a control community.

The intervention consisted of public education activities (e.g. publicising local smoking control plans, organisation of Quit and Win contests), encouraging interventions by health professionals (e.g. training doctors and dentists in cessation methods), work-site activities (e.g. holding smoking-policy workshops and dispensing self-help materials) and developing cessation resources (e.g. maintaining a local smoking resources guide). A total of 58 activities were mandated as part of the intervention, and each intervention community could add their own initiatives (e.g. mass media cessation campaigns). The main aim was to utilise existing resources within each community, but an additional $220,000 per year for 4 years was provided to each intervention community.

For the purposes of evaluation, a smoker was defined as someone (aged 25–64 years) who had smoked at least 100 cigarettes and who was smoking at the time of the initial baseline survey, with a heavy smoker being a smoker of at least 25 cigarettes per day. Approximately 550 heavy and 550 light-moderate smokers were identified in each community and this cohort was followed-up by telephone interview annually from 1988 to 1993 in order to assess the impact of the intervention. The total cohort sample consisted of approximately 5,000 initial heavy smokers (median daily consumption=30) and 5,000 initial light-moderate smokers (median daily consumption=15) in both the intervention and control conditions.

Changes in smoking prevalence and overall quit ratios were also assessed by telephone interviews with over 100,000 households for the baseline survey (1988) and over 50,000 households for the final prevalence survey (1993).

The results of this study were disappointing. Within the heavy smoker cohort, 18.0% in the intervention communities had quit (self-report of no smoking in previous 6 months) by the end of the study, compared with 18.7% in the control communities. For light-moderate smokers the corresponding quit rates were 30.6% and 27.5%, suggesting that the intervention resulted in an extra 3% quitting within this group of smokers. The intervention had no significant impact on total smoking prevalence in either group (falling by just under 3% in all groups) and the overall quit ratio was similar within intervention and control communities.

The detailed results of this trial are worth closer inspection by anyone considering implementing this type of intervention. They suggest that in countries or communities in which the health educational message about smoking is already widely accepted and motivation to quit is generally high, further motivational interventions produce rather small effects and may have absolutely no influence at all on heavy (highly addicted) smokers. It is possible that if a similar intervention had been carried out in a country at a less advanced stage of anti-smoking policy development then it would have had a larger effect, at least among lighter smokers. This is supported by the fact that virtually all of the intervention effect on light-moderate smokers in the COMMIT trial occurred in those with no college education, a portion of the US population which may not have been reached by previous health educational efforts.

One clear implication here is that efforts to increase motivation to quit among addicted smokers may be fairly ineffectual unless accompanied by greater availability of treatments directed at their dependence on nicotine.

Brief smoking cessation interventions by health professionals

Brief advice and encouragement to stop smoking by a health professional during a routine consultation has been recognised to be a particularly cost-effective method of increasing the number of smokers who stop smoking[18]. For example, the GP could briefly advise the smoker in the following way:

> The best thing you can do for your health is to stop smoking and I want to advise you to stop as soon as possible. I know it can be hard and many try several times before finally succeeding. I'd like you to take home this leaflet and read it. It provides some information on the health effects of smoking and some tips on ways of stopping smoking. The sooner you stop the better.

A recent review of the effectiveness of smoking cessation interventions[18] concluded that each episode of systematically applied brief family doctors' advice results in an extra 2% of smokers becoming long-term abstainers (over and above the natural background quit rate). One of the most influential studies on this issue in the UK was that published by Russell and colleagues in 1979[19]. This study randomly allocated all 2,138 smokers attending 28 family doctors in May 1974 to receive either: (a) brief advice (one or two minutes) to stop smoking plus a 4-page leaflet entitled *How you can give up smoking*; (b) brief advice only; (c) a smoking questionnaire only; or (d) no intervention (control group). The proportion of subjects who were abstinent at both one month and one year follow-ups in those groups were: (a) 5.1%; (b) 3.3%; (c) 1.6%; and (d) 0.3%. It was argued that if all the GPs in the UK routinely provided brief advice and a leaflet to smokers then this would produce an extra half million ex-smokers each year.

The intervention in this study worked by motivating more people to try to stop smoking rather than increasing the success rate among those who did try. There was also good evidence that those who succeeded in stopping smoking in that study were generally the lighter smokers. For example, the one year abstainers averaged only 9 cigarettes per day at baseline, compared with 17 per day in those who were still smoking at one month follow-up.

In 1983, Russell and colleagues published another similar study[20] (conducted in November 1980). On this occasion patients were randomly allocated to: (a) no intervention; (b) brief advice plus a booklet; or (c) brief advice plus a booklet plus the offer of nicotine gum. The proportions who were abstinent at both the 4 and 12 month follow-ups were: (a) 3.9%; (b) 4.1%; and (c) 8.8%. Unlike the original study,

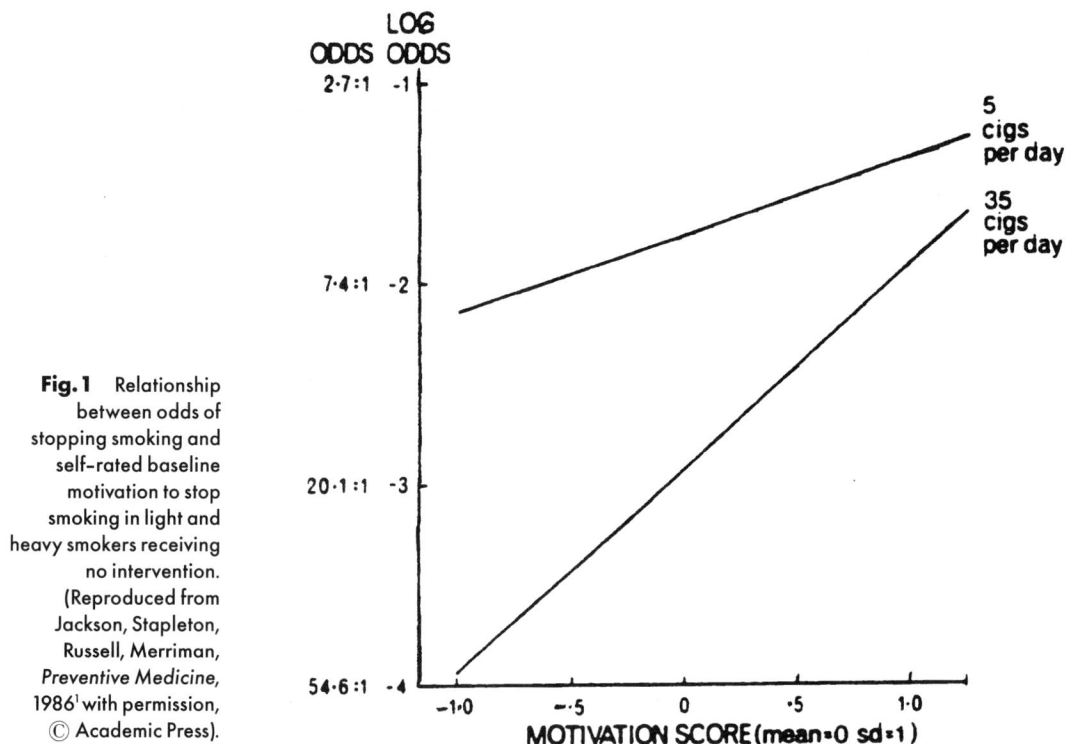

Fig. 1 Relationship between odds of stopping smoking and self-rated baseline motivation to stop smoking in light and heavy smokers receiving no intervention. (Reproduced from Jackson, Stapleton, Russell, Merriman, *Preventive Medicine*, 1986[1] with permission, © Academic Press).

this one found no material effect of brief advice by the family doctor. The reasons for this are not entirely clear, but it is possible that the relative effectiveness of simple brief advice to quit lessened over the six and a half years between the studies, as the general anti-smoking climate within the UK population strengthened. In this study the nicotine gum (provided free) motivated more smokers to try to stop, increased the success rate among those who tried, and reduced the relapse rate of those who stopped.

Subsequent analyses of the results of this study uncovered some interesting relationships between, motivation to quit, tobacco dependence (both assessed pretreatment), and smoking cessation following various family doctor interventions[1]. Figures 1 and 2 illustrate these relationships. Figure 1 shows the relationship between likelihood of successful cessation and strength of motivation to quit in heavy (e.g. 30 cigarettes per day) and light smokers (e.g. 5 per day) receiving no intervention. Heavy smokers are less likely to quit on their own than lighter smokers, but this effect is particularly strong at lower levels of motivation. Thus for a heavy smoker to succeed in stopping smoking they must have a particularly strong desire to quit. Figure 2 illustrates the relationship between gender, tobacco dependence, treatment, and

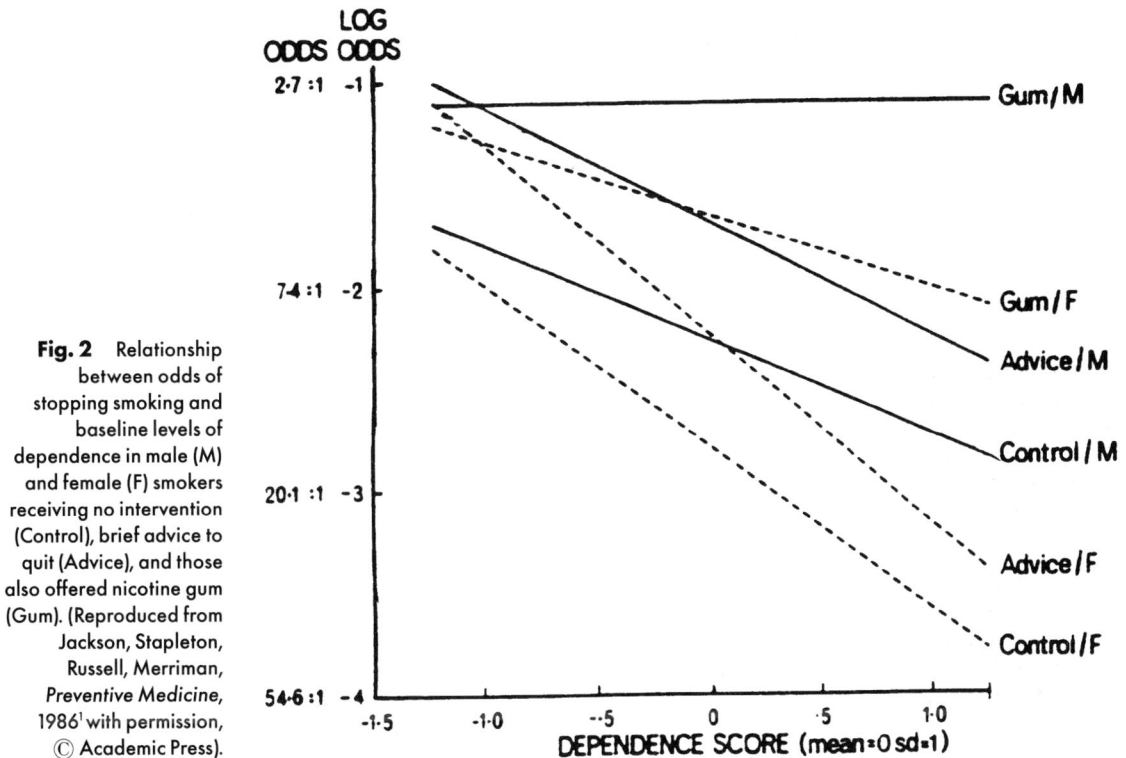

Fig. 2 Relationship between odds of stopping smoking and baseline levels of dependence in male (M) and female (F) smokers receiving no intervention (Control), brief advice to quit (Advice), and those also offered nicotine gum (Gum). (Reproduced from Jackson, Stapleton, Russell, Merriman, *Preventive Medicine*, 1986[1] with permission, © Academic Press).

smoking cessation. More dependent smokers are less likely to quit, but are particularly helped by the offer of nicotine gum. The negative effect of increased dependence appears to be particularly strong in women.

More recently the efficacy of transdermal nicotine patches when used as an accompaniment to family doctors' advice and follow-up has been confirmed in large placebo-controlled trials[12,21]. The results of one such study[12] are illustrated in Figure 3. Consistent with the results of the trial of nicotine gum discussed above, these results indicate that nicotine patches can roughly double the 1-year abstinence rate in motivated and dependent smokers (from about 5% to about 10% 1-year sustained abstinence).

These studies have also suggested that the vast majority of smokers who are going to succeed in quitting following a brief intervention with nicotine patches achieve abstinence within the first week of quitting. Much of the concern about reimbursing for nicotine replacement products or subsidising them on the National Health Service centres around the potentially high cost of providing these products free for months to the vast number of smokers who may wish to use them. The existing evidence suggests that it may be appropriate for a doctor to

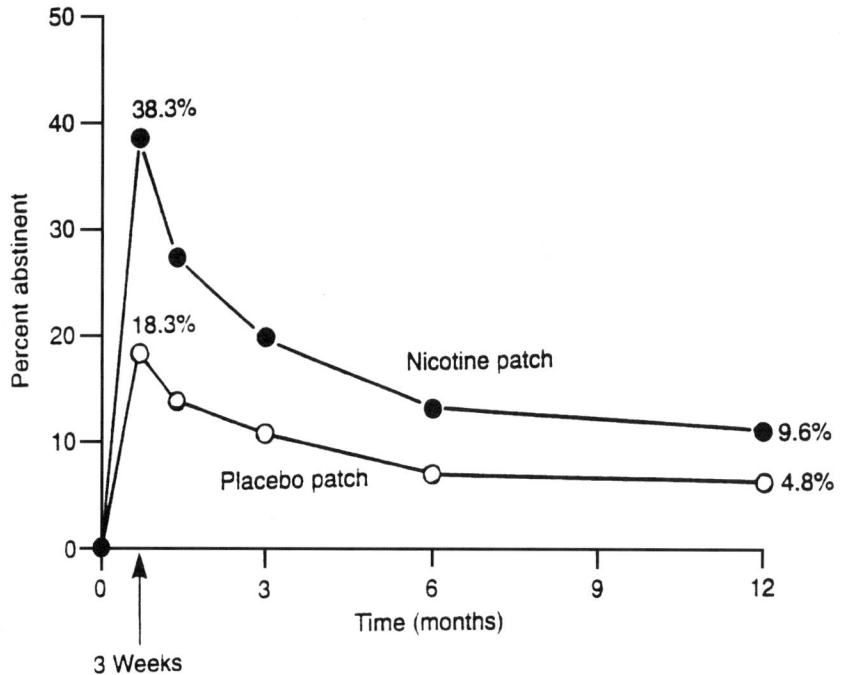

Fig. 3 Continuous abstinence from smoking in patients treated with nicotine patches and placebo patches, combined with brief advice and follow-ups in general practice. (Reproduced from Stapleton, Russell, Feyerabend et al. Addiction, 1995[12] with permission, © Society for the Study of Addiction to Alcohol and other Drugs).

continue to prescribe nicotine replacement only to those who managed to achieve abstinence using the product within the first week. If this became normal practice then it would drastically reduce the potential cost of subsidising nicotine replacement, and would ensure that this medication was being targeted efficiently at those who benefit from it.

A brief treatment intervention for moderate to heavy smokers (i.e. at least 10 cigarettes per day) with some interest in stopping smoking should include the arrangement of a quit date, offer of nicotine replacement medication with advice on its use, and the offer of a follow-up appointment within 1 week of the quit date. Those attending the follow-up and claiming abstinence (ideally confirmed by an afternoon measure of expired carbon-monoxide less than 10 ppm) should be continued on the nicotine replacement according to the recommended treatment schedule (or until they relapse).

Much of the research on brief smoking interventions has focused on interventions by medical doctors. However, it is possible that such interventions would be as effective if carried out by other professionals, such as nurses and pharmacists. Now that nicotine replacement products are available over the pharmacy counter in many countries (i.e. without a doctor's prescription), there is a good case for evaluating the role of the pharmacist as a smoking cessation advisor.

Specialist smoking cessation treatment

The previous sections have outlined the role of public health campaigns and brief interventions by healthcare workers to promote smoking cessation. Such interventions are generally designed to encourage smokers to quit on their own, or to provide a level of clinical help for patients to stop smoking which can be fitted into the routine work of healthcare workers. There is little doubt that, when such interventions are appropriately targeted, they are cost-effective methods of reducing the number of smokers and producing a substantial health gain. However, consistent use of such measures will still leave a large number of smokers who have tried to quit on their own, and tried again following some brief advice from their doctor but without success. This select group of highly motivated and highly addicted smokers are the appropriate clientele for a specialist smokers clinic.

The specific treatment components used in a smokers clinic vary from clinic to clinic. The efficacy of specific components of intensive treatments have generally not been evaluated properly. One is, therefore, forced to select treatment components which have face-validity and some supporting data, as well as components which have been proven effective. Some of the assessment and treatment components which can be advocated for smokers clinics are described below:

Nicotine replacement: Just as nicotine replacement has been shown to be effective as part of a brief intervention, this treatment component has been shown to roughly double long term abstinence rates (e.g. from 16% to 27% when nicotine gum or patch are provided[23]) in the context of an intensive smokers clinic treatment[22-24]. A specialist clinic has the advantage of being able to acquire expertise in the use of nicotine replacement products and can provide a level of support necessary to ensure adequate compliance. Although the nicotine patch is ideal for brief interventions, in that it is relatively easy to use and has a favourable side-effect profile, some of the other nicotine replacement products require more guidance. For example, patients should be advised how to chew nicotine gum in a manner which will enhance buccal absorption and should be prepared for the initial irritant side-effects. Similarly, compliance with nicotine nasal spray treatment may be poor unless provided along with considerable encouragement and explanation (due to initial nasal irritancy).

At the time of writing two strengths of nicotine gum, a variety of transdermal patches (both daytime and 24 h varieties), and a nasal spray are licensed and available in the UK, with new products (e.g. a nicotine inhaler) under evaluation. There is no doubt that these treatments help reduce nicotine withdrawal symptoms and increase the chances of long

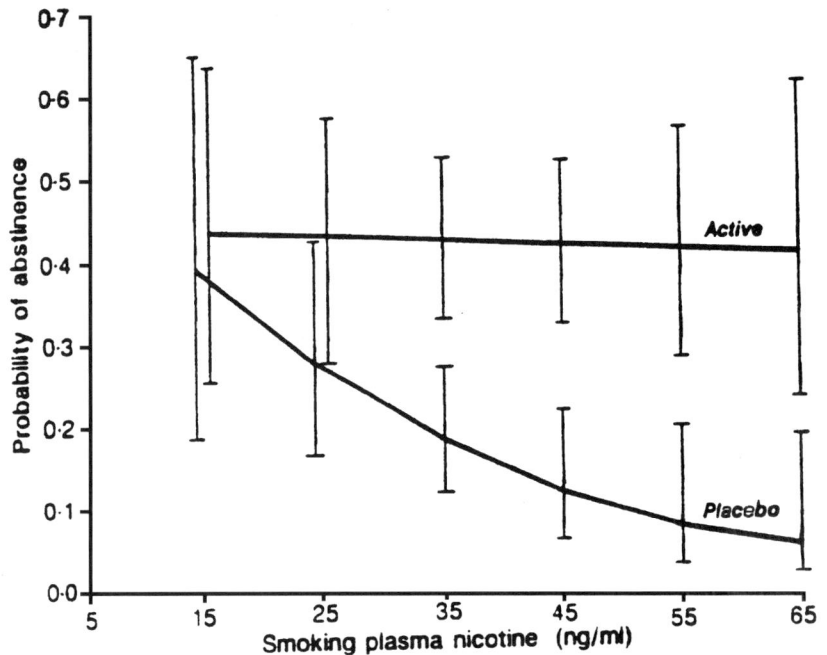

Fig. 4 Relationship between treatment (nicotine or placebo spray), pretreatment smoking plasma nicotine concentration, and abstinence at 3 months (with 95% confidence intervals). (From Sutherland, Stapleton, Russell et al., Randomised controlled trial of nasal nicotine spray in smoking cessation, Lancet 1992; 340: 324-29[24], © by The Lancet Ltd, 1992, with permission).

term abstinence from tobacco. There is also preliminary evidence that certain products are particularly helpful to certain types of smoker. For example, Figure 4 shows the 3 month abstinence rates in subjects attending a smokers clinic and participating in a placebo-controlled trial of nasal nicotine spray[24]. Among those receiving placebo spray, the heavier their nicotine intake while smoking prior to the trial (as assessed by baseline blood nicotine concentration) the less likely they were to be abstinent at 3 months follow-up. This relationship was completely offset in those who received the nicotine spray. One can therefore see that the nasal spray was particularly helpful to the heaviest smokers, producing an 8-fold increase in their chances of achieving abstinence from cigarettes.

Preliminary evidence suggests that combining nicotine replacement products (e.g. patch plus gum) can enhance abstinence rates[25] and again this is the type of treatment which could best be offered in a specialist clinic.

Group treatment: By recruiting clients from a wide geographical area, smokers clinics can provide regular group treatments, and so benefit from this more efficient use of therapist time. Stop-smoking groups aim to provide additional support in order to help maintain abstinence in the first month during which most relapse occurs, and to encourage the use of positive smoking cessation strategies (e.g. proper use of nicotine replacement products, avoidance of high-risk relapse situations, etc.). There is also some evidence that the use of group processes can actually enhance both attendance and abstinence rates[26]. The clinician can encourage therapeutic group processes by increasing group cohesion (e.g. by asking group members to introduce themselves, initiating group discussions, etc.) and enhancing group pressure to maintain abstinence (e.g. by initiating publicly declared commitments to remain abstinent).

Biochemical feedback on smoke intake: There are now a number of methods of biochemically quantifying patients' smoke intake[27]. Saliva cotinine is the 'gold standard' measure (for individuals not using nicotine replacement) and can be measured accurately in samples sent to a laboratory by post[28]. Expired carbon monoxide (CO) monitors are now widely available and have the advantage of providing an immediate quantitative feedback of the amount of smoke which the patient has recently inhaled. Expired CO is about 90% accurate in discriminating a smoker from a nonsmoker[27]. There is some evidence that the use of this measure at assessment and follow-up encourages more smokers in disadvantaged socioeconomic groups to quit[29] and it may facilitate the cohesiveness of groups due to greater confidence of honest self-reporting by the participants. Portable CO monitors for use with smokers cost around £450, and there is a good case for these being used routinely in hospital clinics and general practice. However, this assessment and treatment tool is currently only used routinely in specialist clinics.

Unfortunately, other than nicotine replacement, none of these (or any other) treatment components have been adequately evaluated. Perhaps the best guide to the kind of long term results produced by an intensive smokers clinic treatment combining these and other components can be gained from analysis of the results of the Lung Health Study[30] in the US. This study is therefore described in some detail below.

The Lung Health Study (LHS)

This landmark study aimed to assess whether an intensive smoking cessation intervention and the use of a bronchodilator could slow the rate of decline in lung function in otherwise healthy smokers who already had mild impairment of lung function. 5,887 smokers, aged 35–60 years, were randomly allocated to receive either: (1) smoking intervention plus bronchodilator; (2) smoking intervention plus placebo; or (3) no intervention. All participants smoked at least 10 cigarettes per day, were willing to consider smoking cessation, and to participate in a 5-year follow-up. In practice the group averaged 31 cigarettes per day and had smoked for 31 years. Thus all the participants in this study were moderate to heavy smokers with moderate to high motivation to stop smoking.

Because a major aim of the study was to assess the effect of smoking cessation on lung function (and therefore required a high proportion of participants to successfully quit), the investigators used an intensive intervention which could reasonably be considered 'state of the art' at the time the trial was designed. 3,923 subjects were randomised to receive the smoking intervention and 1,964 to receive usual care. The smoking intervention involved 12 group meetings within the first 10 weeks (4 meetings in the first week), with the quit day set at the beginning of the programme. Within the groups, emphasis was placed on behaviour modification techniques and expired CO was measured at every appointment. Relapse prevention skills were taught and relapsers were able to restart treatment immediately (throughout the 5-year duration of the study). Spouses and significant others were included in the cessation programme if they wished, and follow-up appointments were arranged every 4 months. Nicotine replacement therapy (nicotine gum) was used 'aggressively' and provided free to all participants throughout the trial.

This intensive intervention was rewarded by cessation rates amongst the highest reported in a major trial. 35% of the intervention group were abstinent at 1 year (compared with 9% in the no-intervention control group) and 22% of the intervention group sustained abstinence for 5 years (compared with 5% of the control group). These results provide some indication of what impact an intensive treatment provided at a smokers clinic can have compared with the natural background cessation rate occurring as a result of health education, usual care by healthcare workers and naturally occurring self-quit attempts.

The stepped care approach: implications for clinical practice

Ideally, each smoker should be targeted with the least expensive treatment which is likely to enable that person to stop smoking. This requires matching the intensity of the intervention to the smoker's levels of motivation and addiction. This paper has described four steps or levels of intervention, each of which is appropriate for smokers with particular levels of motivation and addiction. These are summarised below:

1. The first level of intervention involves the provision of health education and other such information designed to increase motivation to quit

smoking. This type of intervention can be delivered relatively cheaply to the population via the mass media. It should be targeted at sections of the population not yet aware of the information provided (those with little current desire to stop smoking).

2. The next level is the provision of brief (i.e. lasting a couple of minutes at most) advice to stop smoking from health professionals. In populations which have not already been saturated with such messages, both of these first two levels of intervention can result in more people making an attempt to stop smoking, with a worthwhile number (of mainly light smokers) actually succeeding in becoming long term abstainers. Those with moderate levels of motivation and addiction should be offered more help.

3. The next level of intervention is for healthcare workers to offer nicotine replacement plus a follow-up appointment. This type of intervention might require a total of about 20 min of the clinician's time. It increases the proportion who try to quit, but also the proportion who actually succeed. Such interventions are able to help moderately motivated and addicted smokers to quit.

4. Finally, one has the intensive treatments which can most appropriately be offered in a specialist clinic. Such interventions are relatively expensive per smoker treated, but, if based on treatment in groups, may still be cost effective due to higher success rates (group treatment requires an average of about 30 min therapist time per patient). Unlike the less expensive interventions, intensive support with nicotine replacement helps the more highly addicted smokers to quit (i.e. those who are destined to suffer the greatest health consequences).

More detailed descriptions of the application of the stepped care approach in medical settings have been proposed[31]. It has been suggested that about 20% of smokers might appropriately be treated with nicotine replacement and brief support (level 3), and about 5% with nicotine replacement and intensive support (level 4).

In many countries (including the UK), virtually all the smoking cessation resources have been targeted at the first two levels of intervention. GPs have been encouraged to shoulder much of the burden for encouraging smokers to quit, but neither they nor their staff are usually provided with resources (e.g. a CO monitor, ability to prescribe subsidised nicotine replacement) or training in implementing effective smoking cessation interventions. Recent trials of very brief interventions on smoking (health checks by practice nurses) do not support the effectiveness of this intervention[32].

In countries in which public desire to stop smoking is already high, there is a need to meet that demand with some form of treatment for those who have been unable to do so on their own. This may be particularly the case for the more deprived sections of society. 22% of UK social classes I and II are smokers (64% of whom want to stop), and 55% are ex-smokers. Among the unemployed, 55% are smokers (67% of whom want to stop) and only 20% are ex-smokers. Around 80% of smokers in both social groups have already tried unsuccessfully to quit. Thus it seems as though the current higher smoking rate in the poorer sections of society is due to a difficulty in stopping smoking once an attempt has been made rather than a lack of desire to quit[33]. Compared with treatment services for other addictions, there is a marked absence of provision of specialist smoking cessation services. Given the vast health consequences and addictiveness of tobacco smoking there is a good case for every large general hospital having its own specialist smoking cessation service, to provide intensive treatment for highly motivated and addicted smokers, and to train and support other healthcare workers to deliver brief interventions as part of their routine work.

Acknowledgements

The support of Merton Sutton and Wandsworth Health Authority is gratefully acknowledged. Thanks for support and helpful comments are owed to Professor MAH Russell, Mr MJ Jarvis, Dr R West and Professor HA Ghodse.

References

1 Jackson PH, Stapleton JA, Russell MAH, Merriman RJ. Predictors of outcome in a general practitioner intervention against smoking. *Prev Med* 1986; **15**: 244–53
2 Sanders D, Peveler R, Mant D, Fowler G. Predictors of successful smoking cessation following advice from nurses in general practice. *Addiction* 1993; **88**: 1699–705
3 DiClemente CC, Prochaska JO, Fairhurst SK, Velicer WF, Velasquez MM, Rossi JS. The process of smoking cessation: an analysis of precontemplation, contemplation and preparation stages of change. *J Consult Clin Psychol* 1991; **59**: 294–304
4 Prochaska JO, DiClemente CC, Velicier W, Rossi JS. Standardised, individualised, interactive and personalised self-help programs for smoking cessation. *Health Psychol* 1993; **12**: 394–405
5 US Department of Health and Human Services. *The Health Consequences of Smoking: Nicotine Addiction*. Washington DC: US Government Printing Office. 1988
6 Hughes JR, Gulliver S, Fenwick JW *et al*. Smoking cessation among self-quitters. *Health Psychol* 1992; **11**: 331–34
7 Cohen S, Lichtenstein E, Prochaska JO *et al*. Debunking myths about self-quitting: evidence from 10 prospective studies of persons who attempt to quit smoking by themselves. *Am Psychol* 1989; **11**: 1355–65
8 American Psychiatric Association. *Diagnostic and Statistical Manual of Mental Disorders* (4th edn). Washington DC. 1994
9 Hughes JR. Tobacco withdrawal in self-quitters. *J Consult Clin Psychol* 1992; **60**: 689–97
10 Hughes JR, Gust SW, Skoog K, Keenan R, Fenwick JW. Symptoms of tobacco withdrawal: a replication and extension. *Arch Gen Psychiatry* 1991; **48**: 52–9

11 Heatherton TF, Kozlowski LT, Frecker RC, Fagerstrom KO. The Fagerstrom test for nicotine dependence: a revision of the Fagerstrom tolerance questionnaire. *Br J Addiction* 1991; **86**: 1119–27

12 Stapleton JA, Russell MAH, Feyerabend C *et al*. Dose effects and predictors of outcome in a randomised trial of nicotine patches in general practice. *Addiction* 1995; **90**: 31–42

13 Puska P, Salonen JT, Nissinen A *et al*. Change in risk factors for coronary heart disease during 10 years of a community intervention programme (North Karelia project). *BMJ* 1983; **287**: 1840–4

14 Fortmann SP, Taylor CB, Flora JA, Jatulis DE. Changes in adult cigarette smoking after 5 years of community health education: the Stanford five-city project. *Am J Epidemiol* 1993; **137**: 82–96

15 Lando HA, Pechacek TF, Pirie PL *et al*. Changes in cigarette smoking in the Minnesota Heart Health Program. *Am J Public Health* 1995; **85**: 201–8

16 The COMMIT Research Group. Community Intervention Trial for Smoking Cessation (COMMIT): I. Cohort results from a four-year community intervention. *Am J Public Health* 1995; **85**: 183–92

17 The COMMIT Research Group. Community Intervention Trial for Smoking Cessation (COMMIT): II. Changes in adult cigarette smoking prevalence. *Am J Public Health* 1995; **85**: 193–200

18 Law M, Tang JL, Wald N. An analysis of the effectiveness of interventions intended to help people stop smoking. *Arch Intern Med* 1995; **155**: 1933–41

19 Russell MAH, Wilson C, Taylor C, Baker CD. Effect of general practitioners' advice against smoking. *BMJ* 1979; **ii**: 231–5

20 Russell MAH, Merriman R, Stapleton J, Taylor W. Effect of nicotine chewing gum as an adjunct to general practitioners' advice against smoking. *BMJ* 1983; **287**: 1782–5

21 Imperial Cancer Research Fund General Practice Research Group. Effectiveness of a nicotine patch in helping people stop smoking: results of a randomised trial in general practice. *BMJ* 1993; **306**: 1304–8

22 Foulds J. Does nicotine replacement therapy work? *Addiction* 1993; **88**: 1473–8

23 Silagy C, Mant D, Fowler G, Lodge M. Meta-analysis on the efficacy of nicotine replacement therapies in smoking cessation. *Lancet* 1994; **343**: 139–42

24 Sutherland G, Stapleton J, Russell MAH *et al*. Randomised controlled trial of nasal nicotine spray in smoking cessation. *Lancet* 1992; **340**: 324–9

25 Kornitzer M, Boutsen M, Dramaix M, Thijs J, Gustavsson G. Combined use of nicotine patch and gum in smoking cessation: a placebo-controlled clinical trial. *Prev Med* 1995; **24**: 41–7

26 Hajek P, Belcher M, Stapleton J. Enhancing the impact of groups: an evaluation of two group formats for smokers. *Br J Clin Psychol* 1985; **24**: 289–94

27 Jarvis MJ, Tunstall-Pedoe H, Feyerabend C, Vesey C, Saloojee Y. Comparison of tests used to distinguish smokers from nonsmokers. *Am J Public Health* 1987; **77**: 1435–8

28 Foulds J, Bryant A, Stapleton J, Jarvis MJ, Russell MAH. The stability of cotinine in unfrozen saliva mailed to the laboratory. *Am J Public Health* 1994; **84**: 1182–3

29 Jamrozik K, Vessey M, Fowler G *et al*. Controlled trial of three different antismoking interventions in general practice. *BMJ* 1984; **288**: 1499–503

30 Anthonisen NR, Connet JE, Kiley JP *et al*. for the Lung Health Study Research Group. Effects of smoking intervention and the use of inhaled anticholinergic bronchodilator on the rate of decline of FEV1: The Lung Health Study. *JAMA* 1994; **272**: 1497–505

31 Foulds J, Jarvis MJ. Smoking cessation and prevention. In Calverley P, Pride N, eds. *Chronic Obstructive Pulmonary Disease*. London: Chapman and Hall, 1995: 373–90

32 Imperial Cancer Research Fund OXCHECK Study Group. Effectiveness of health checks conducted by nurses in primary care: final results of the OXCHECK study. *BMJ* 1995; **310**: 1099–104

33 West R. *The Nicotine Trap: a Report on Smoking Cessation in the UK*. London: Health Education Authority, 1995

Forty years on: a war to recognise and win

How the tobacco industry has survived the revelations on smoking and health

David Pollock

Formerly Director, Action on Smoking and Health

Nothing has significantly checked the growth of the tobacco industry since the introduction of smoking to Europe, and the industry has easily survived the 40 years since the first authoritative revelations about the health effects of smoking. Some explanations are offered and the tactics of the industry and the response of the UK Government are reviewed. The policies of British–American Tobacco and its subsidiaries, especially Brown and Williamson in the USA, are considered in detail, including the rejection of an early proposal for a pragmatic but honest deal. In particular, an internal document from 1970 is examined in which BAT purports to set policy for the whole industry. The document is revealed as showing far-sighted but cynical calculation, for instance, in limiting concessions to those countries where public and government awareness requires them. Examples of BAT activities are quoted to illustrate key points.

The tobacco industry is an egregious example of mankind's failure to control the market and of the market's failure to serve the true interests of mankind. It is also, regrettably, one of the few industries—another is arms—where the UK is a major player on the world scene: BAT alone has tobacco subsidiaries in 49 countries and through them supplies 10.6%[1] of the world market, just behind Philip Morris's 12%[2]. It is on BAT that I wish to concentrate in this article, drawing on various documents that have recently come to light, mainly in the USA.

Tobacco was a special commodity from the time it was first brought to Europe in the fifteenth century. James I, who (anonymously but famously) railed against it[3], soon found that he could not eliminate 'this vile custome of **Tobacco** taking' whether by persuasion or by punitive taxation and instead became hooked on the income it provided[4]. Elsewhere, papal bans and Japanese imperial edicts[5] were equally powerless, while the fiscal potential motivated the creation of state monopolies in many European kingdoms which are only now being dismantled.

But the modern industry was not born until James Duke leased and installed two of James Bonsack's newly invented cigarette-making machines in 1884, each doing the work of 30–40 hand-rollers[6].

Present address: David Pollock, 13 Dunsmure Road, London N16 5PU, UK

Mechanisation led in short order to the emergence of significant enterprises, including W Duke, Sons & Co and R J Reynolds Tobacco Company in the USA and Imperial Tobacco in the UK. In the 1890s James Duke created the monopolistic American Tobacco trust which, not content with 90% of total US sales, invaded the British market too. Imperial's counterattack in the US led in 1902 to a truce: each kept out of the other's home market while they created the jointly owned British-American Tobacco Company to exploit their brands in the rest of the world. Anti-trust litigation led in 1911 to the break-up of American Tobacco, which was forced to sell its interest in BAT. Now wholly British, BAT was free to enter the American market in competition with its former parent. In 1927 it bought the US company Brown and Williamson, and in 1994 the American Tobacco Company, successor of its former parent, giving it about 19% of the US market[7]. To this day, however, BAT has almost no presence in the British market.

The world market for tobacco is dominated by a handful of hugely profitable US and British companies, which have a controlling presence not only in all western countries but throughout the third world. Since 1989 they have bought up most of the industry in the former communist world, with BAT making major acquisitions, for example, in Hungary, Ukraine, Uzbekistan, Russia and Poland[8]. The exception is China, but even that bastion of state monopoly seems doomed to fall: Beijing has agreed under American pressure to allow imports to compete with the Chinese National Tobacco Company, the largest company of all: its domestic market alone makes up about one-third of total world sales. Hitherto more used to allocation and distribution than to marketing and sales, CNTC will either have to learn the ruthless ways of its western rivals or succumb: Philip Morris is already advertising there in anticipation of the market opening, and BAT's 1994 annual report writes ominously of China's 'longer term business potential'.

How is it that this industry has not only survived for 40 years the apparently devastating revelations about the risks of smoking but is still flourishing and expanding? It is a sobering fact that more disease and death have been generated by smoking **since** the health consequences became known than in all the previous history of tobacco use. Other companies, faced with revelations about health risks that are negligible by comparison, hasten to publish warning advertisements and withdraw offending products from the market. When Perrier found its water was contaminated with minute traces of benzene, millions of bottles were called in and tipped away. A cigarette boasts far more benzene and a cocktail of dozens of other carcinogens and poisons besides.

The asbestos industry has collapsed under the weight of regulation and litigation, almost bringing down the Lloyds insurance market with it; the nuclear power industry in many countries has been brought to its knees by public protest about health risks barely measurable on the same scale as those from smoking. Not so the tobacco companies. What has allowed them to continue killing their customers with apparent impunity?

Extrinsic factors have helped. When the problems emerged, the rule of *caveat emptor* was still strong and the consumer movement in its infancy. Disbelief affected even some doctors that so accepted a habit could be a killer. The extent of the risk was underestimated and even so the politicians sought to avoid panic. Iain Macleod, the Minister of Health, told the Cabinet in 1954 that he would accompany his Parliamentary statement about the presumptively causal relationship between smoking and lung cancer with a Lobby conference when he would encourage the press 'to maintain a due sense of proportion'[9]. The long delay between starting smoking and the onset of disease facilitated (as it still does) ignorant or wilful mockery of the connection. These doubts promoted 'denial' by smokers, intent on feeding their addiction, and prevarication by the companies, intent on milking it for the maximum profit.

Indeed, it was in no-one's interest to destroy the industry. It curtailed smokers' cravings, provided lucrative careers to its managers, made huge profits for its shareholders, and paid immense taxes to governments. The British Government was naively wary of precipitating a collapse in sales: Chancellor of the Exchequer Peter Thorneycroft warned a Cabinet committee in 1957 of 'the enormous contribution to the Exchequer from tobacco duties and the serious effect on the Commonwealth, in particular on Rhodesia, that a campaign against smoking would have'[10]. And crucially the victims, unlike those of asbestos or nuclear power, could be blamed for their own fate — a line adopted from the start by the British Government[11] and ruthlessly followed by the industry, which still denies that nicotine is addictive even though as long ago as 1963 BAT was told in an expert report that it 'appears to be intimately connected with the phenomena of tobacco habituation (tolerance) and/or addiction'[12].

The companies from the start adopted tactics designed to protect their shareholders' investments. In the UK, the industry offered the Government £250,000 (worth about £3.6 million today) for research: the Cabinet minutes reveal that some Ministers thought it improper to accept what amounted to a bribe, but most were keen to take the cash[13]. In the USA the notorious Frank Statement of false reassurance to smokers was published and the Council for Tobacco Research was formed as a public relations gambit. Driven by the structural imperatives of a public company, even scientists with moral doubts about their actions were swept along in a strategy that switched from seeking, in the 1950s, to disprove the health charge to trying, in the 1960s, to limit the harmful constituents and then, in the 1970s, to producing synthetic smoking materials and so-called safe cigarettes. When these efforts failed, research turned to serving the marketing efforts of a new generation of hardheaded managers intent on resisting controls as long as possible and maximising profits in the meantime[14]. This transition was marked by the formation, in 1979, of the International Committee on Smoking Issues (ICOSI) (later called Infotab and now the Tobacco Documentation Centre) which helped the western companies concert across the world their public line on health and tobacco control issues, for example by producing tendentious model answers to awkward questions about smoking and health or about companies' different standards in developed and developing countries.

By then the industry was trapped in a policy — which continues to this day — of arrogant denial of known facts and careless disregard for customers' welfare while extracting the maximum short-term profit. Though always a likely outcome, it was not inevitable. Once any lingering doubt about the risks of smoking vanished from the minds of the industry bosses, they might have sought a pragmatic deal with governments to limit their liability for past damage (litigation by smokers began in the USA in the mid-1950s) in return for a rapid switch to less dangerous products.

Something on these lines was indeed proposed by Addison Yeaman, Brown & Williamson's top in-house lawyer, in 1963[15]. Alarmed at the threat posed by the Surgeon-General's imminent (first) report, he seized on the finding in BAT's research report that nicotine had a 'tranquillizing' function ('nicotine, an addictive drug effective in the release of stress mechanisms') and a 'possible effect on obesity' and on (exaggerated) expectations of work on cigarette filters by a B&W scientist, Dr RB Griffith[16].

In these, Yeaman saw an opportunity for the industry to 'pass from its present terrain of defense to a field for effective counter attack'. He proposed putting these allegedly beneficial effects of smoking and the safeguard of the filters in the balance against the health risks certain to be publicised by the Surgeon-General's report. Simultaneously B&W should commission, in cooperation (he proposed) with the Surgeon-General, the American Cancer Society and others, 'massive and impressively financed research' into smoking and health, conducted through a 'new organization' that was 'autonomous . . . uncontrolled'; and the industry should 'steel itself to issuing a warning', thereby reinforcing the defence argument in product liability suits that the plaintiffs had voluntarily assumed the risks. Yeaman's approach was not intended as a surrender — indeed, he saw competitive advantage for B&W in it — but it was too radical and risky for B&W and was rejected. Thereafter he kept to the orthodox line.

A few years later, B&W's parent company BAT can be seen in a leaked document[17] at a defining moment in its policy on smoking and health. A 1970 paper, addressed to the chiefs of all its associated companies, sets out an approach that owes a great deal more to commercial considerations than to concern for health. It says that BAT, 'the largest tobacco company in the world', should wherever possible 'exercise leadership within the industry on the question of Smoking and Health' in the face of 'the growing threat to the industry in a number of countries . . . that its operations will be seriously restricted by legislation'. BAT saw itself as giving a lead away from attitudes in other companies that are 'through their intransigence likely to provoke the legislation we seek to avoid'.

BAT's 'over-riding policy' was, therefore, 'to discourage and delay the process of restrictive legislative action by governments in every way possible' — allegedly to allow more time for research (work on artificial smoking materials was just beginning). The policy should be to avoid 'unnecessary conflict' with medical authorities which might provoke government action. 'While in the past it has seemed good sense . . . to contest the validity of all the evidence against smoking (and may still be necessary to avoid damages in lawsuits), there is little doubt that the inflexibility of this attitude is beginning to create in some countries hostility and even contempt for the industry among intelligent, fair-minded doctors.' The future line should therefore be that 'as tobacco manufacturers we are not competent to express any authoritative view on a medical matter' but that there is disagreement about the evidence. 'It seems to us that, in the absence of clinical proof of the mechanism involved, causation at the present time remains an open question' and that more research should therefore be undertaken.

This line was generally adopted within the industry[18] and is still on offer 25 years later as a defence against effective tobacco control measures. As BAT's director of research wrote in 1976: 'the public position of tobacco companies . . . is dominated by legal considerations . . . Companies are actively seeking to make products acceptable as safer while denying strenuously the need to do so . . . The industry has retreated behind impossible demands for "scientific proof" whereas such proof has never been required as a basis for action in the legal and political fields'[19].

The BAT 1970 policy paper, recognising that governments could not be completely controlled, admitted that compromises were inevitable 'to maintain the industry's survival and prosperity. Our policy . . . is that negotiation should be pursued to its limits . . . in order to fend off anti-smoking legislation'. A line would need to be concerted between companies in each country where a threat arose, but some general principles are set out in the policy paper. 'Legislation is worse for the industry than self-imposed restraints': voluntary restrictions presented the industry in a more favourable light and might with benefit be offered 'at a significantly earlier stage than the moment when legislation is the only alternative'.

This was plainly the spirit in which the UK companies had adopted their code on tobacco advertising ('this vague and woolly collection of criteria' as a Board of Trade official called it[20]) after the first report of the Royal College of Physicians and it was similarly the spirit in which the year after this document appeared the minimal concessions in the UK's first voluntary agreement on tobacco advertising were offered. The principle is to **seem** to be making concessions while actually giving away nothing of value: as the BAT paper said, 'viewed objectively, it may be less harmful than might be supposed to forfeit the use of one or more of the normal advertising media. It might in certain circumstances not be harmful at all' — if more effective and less provocative methods of promotion (merchandising is given as an example) could be used instead.

The paper suggests as a first step that a voluntary advertising code be agreed (e.g. no health claims, no appeals to the young, etc.) — but **not** in those countries where BAT has a minority market share. There it would be better to 'seek out alternative concessions . . . The publication of tar and nicotine tables seems relatively harmless [and] may indeed be of real help . . . since they give nervous smokers an opportunity to continue to smoke with **what they see** as relative safety' (emphasis added). Accordingly, every BAT company should have a brand at or very near the bottom of tar and nicotine tables. No doubt such brands were promoted as 'milder' and 'lighter', but the document stipulates that if there is to be any suggestion that low-tar cigarettes were actually **safer** 'it must come from the government', not the industry, presumably mainly to avoid the damaging implication that their other brands were less safe but probably also because they already realised that low-tar cigarettes offer dubious health benefits at best[21].

The BAT paper goes so far as to say that if governments laid down maximum tar levels 'such action might be welcome . . . because [it] implies to the public that cigarettes meeting these standards are "safe"'. As to packs, while warnings in small print and 'relatively innocuous' wording could be less harmful than voluntary restrictions on the use of advertising media, printing tar and nicotine levels on packs should be strongly resisted. However, a possible concession to governments would be 'to offer . . . to help finance . . . an advertising campaign advocating moderation in smoking . . . There is little reason to suppose that its effect on total consumption would be drastic . . . but the industry would be recognised by government and the public to be taking a responsible attitude.'

The level of far-sighted cynical calculation revealed in this policy statement has not diminished 25 years later. The industry is pursuing its own best interests, not those of consumers or governments, in a policy characterised by casuistry and bad faith. Despite the plain admissions in his company's files, Sir Patrick Sheehy, chairman of BAT, told his 1990

AGM: 'cigarette smoking has not been proven to cause disease . . . A statistical association does not establish causation. Further research is needed . . .' — and, when pressed, added 'I really do not have any comment . . . none at all. I am not a medical authority'[22] and the chief executive officers of the US companies, including BAT's Brown & Williamson, all swore to a Congress committee in 1994 that nicotine was not in their belief addictive. Despite their assurances that nothing is further from their wishes than that children should smoke, companies pursue the young smoker competitively in advertising and promotional campaigns: BAT's Canadian part-owned subsidiary Imperial Tobacco in its 1988 marketing plan stated: 'if the last ten years have taught us anything, it is that the industry is dominated by the companies who respond most effectively to the needs of younger smokers' — and proceeded to define the 'target groups' for various brands as 'men [aged] 12–17' or 'men and women [aged] 12–34'[23]. Adept use of small concessions in successive voluntary agreements has kept legislative control at bay in the UK[24] and elsewhere.

Similarly, the differentiation of stance from country to country, evident in the 1970 BAT policy paper and thought to require explanation (especially as between developed and developing countries) in some of ICOSI's 1979 model answers, continues to this day. Thus, in 1993, Dr Sharon Boyse, head of BAT's Smoking Issues Department, visited Sri Lanka and reassured smokers that there was 'absolutely no laboratory proof that smoking is directly related to lung cancer or heart disease' — whereas lung cancer could be caused by keeping pet birds. David Bishop, chairman of BAT's local company, deplored the media's failure to highlight all the research that 'paints a different picture from what people have been led to believe all this time'[25]. It is difficult to imagine so deliberate a bullish line being taken in the UK.

Explaining its apparent moderation, the BAT 1970 policy document says: 'in the long run . . . it is likely to be damaging to BAT, and to the industry to act as though a "war" exists between the industry and the government on Smoking and Health. If a "war" exists, or is believed to exist, then it is one which in the end we stand to lose.' Clearer advice to public health advocates could not be found: a bright light must be cast on the ways that the tobacco industry is indeed at war with public health. The cynical promotion of smoking, whether covertly to children in Canada or openly to women in Asia, the denials in public of what has been privately admitted for over 30 years, whether of the health effects of smoking or the addictive qualities of nicotine, and the manipulation of tar tables and of politicians alike — these and all the other trickery the industry relies on for survival worldwide need to be exposed as the acts of war they are. Then and only then will we in the end stand to win.

References and notes

1   *BAT Annual Report* 1994

2   *Philip Morris Annual Report* 1993

3   *A Counter-Blaste to Tobacco* 1603

4   Hill A. ed. *A Counter-Blast to Tobacco*, The Rodale Press, 1954, quoted in Taylor P. *The Smoke Ring*, 2nd edn. London: Sphere, 1985

5   Henningfield JE. *Nicotine — an old-fashioned addiction*. London: Burke, 1985: p 94 sqq

6   Goodman J. *Tobacco in History*. London: Routledge, 1993

7   *Tobacco Reporter*, March 1995: p 12

8   *BAT Annual Report* 1994

9   Cabinet minutes, 10 February 1954

10 Minutes of GEN 588 Cabinet committee, 7 May 1957

11 'The Government should not seek to intrude into the sphere of an individual's personal responsibility. It was, however, important to stress [in a forthcoming statement] this element of personal choice since direct Government action was excluded.' Minutes of Cabinet GEN 588 committee, 3 June 1957

12 Geissbuhler H, Haselbach C. *The Fate of Nicotine in the Body: Report for BAT from Battelle Memorial Institute*. Geneva: unpublished, 1963. This and most of the other company documents quoted in this article have since the time it was prepared been published on the Internet by Prof. Stanton Glantz of the University of California in San Francisco. They can be accessed at http://www.library.ucsf.edu/tobacco/docs/html/xxxx.xx, where the individual document reference number replaces the 'xxxx.xx'. This report is document Ref. 1200.20. The documents are introduced in the first of the series of articles published in a special edition of the *Journal of the American Medical Association* in July 1995 (see Glantz *et al. JAMA* 1995; 274: 219–24)

13 Cabinet minutes 10 February 1954. The calculated use of cash has been taken much further in the USA, but one spectacularly successful example in the UK was the gift (under the voluntary agreement of 1983) of (reportedly) £11 million to fund a Health Promotion Research Trust — provided its work ignored tobacco. The effect was to produce, until the HPRT was wound up in 1993, division and dissension in the health community between those urging a boycott of 'dirty money' and those compelled to accept it if their work was to be funded at all

14 This account is based on unpublished notes in ASH's possession of a journalist's interview in 1981 with Dr SJ Green, then recently retired after about 20 years as research director of BAT

15 Yeoman A. *Implications of Battelle Hippo I & II and the Griffith Filter*. Unpublished paper dated 17 July 1963—Internet Ref. 1802.05 (see Note 12)

16 Just two years later, the same Dr Griffith was to cause alarm on his return from a visit to England when he reported: 'scientists with whom I talked were unanimous in their opinion that smoke is weakly carcinogenic' and that BAT's 'entire laboratory facilities are operating on a 'crash' basis on the smoking and health problem' (report to Brown and Williamson Executive Committee, July 1965)—Internet Ref. 1805.01 (see Note 12)

17 Hargrove GC. *Smoking and Health*. 12 June 1970—Internet Ref. 1186.01 (see Note 12)

18 For example, Sir John Partridge, then chairman of Imperial Tobacco, used it in 1975 at the company's AGM: 'as a company we do not make, indeed we are not qualified to make, medical judgements... As with so many other things where excess of use has a bearing, responsibility must lie with the only person able to exercise control — the consumer'—Internet Ref. 2231.04 (see Note 12)

19 Green SJ. *Cigarette Smoking and Causal Relationships*. 27 October 1976—Internet Ref. 2331.08 (see Note 12). The question of the sufficiency of grounds for action was raised both (a) in the Government's decision in 1957 to remove from a Medical Research Council statement before publication the observation that 'the evidence [about smoking and lung cancer] now available is stronger than that which in comparable matters, is commonly taken as a basis for definite action' (Cabinet committee GEN 588, minutes of 7 May 1957) and (b) in the House of Commons Health Committee's accusation that in rejecting a ban on tobacco advertising the Government was 'awaiting a level of proof about its effectiveness which is in the nature of things

unobtainable' (*Second report, 1992/93: The European Commission's Proposed Directive on the Advertising of Tobacco Products*. London: HMSO, 1992)

20 Public Record Office reference BT 258: 1405. July 1962

21 By 1977, BAT's director of research was asking his chairman: 'should we 'cheat' smokers by 'cheating' League Tables? . . . should we use our superior knowledge of our products to design them so that they give low league table positions but higher deliveries on human smoking?' (Suggested Questions for CAC.III, 26 August 1977)—Internet Ref. 2231.09 (see Note 12)

22 BAT transcript

23 Quoted in *The Nation* 6 May 1991; *The Observer* 10 November 1991. Similarly, in the USA, RJ Reynolds' 'Old Joe Camel' cartoon lifted Camel's share of the under-18 market from 0.5% to 32.8% while leaving the adult share untouched (DiFranza J *et al. RJR Nabisco's cartoon camel promotes Camel cigarettes to children. JAMA* 1991; **266**: 3149–53); while in the UK, the playground humour of Imperial Tobacco's 'Reg' advertising campaign seems to have increased the prevalence of smoking by under-age teenage boys in the areas where it ran, while prevalence was unchanged elsewhere (*An Investigation of the Appeal and Impact of the Embassy Regal 'Reg' Campaign on Young People*. London: Health Education Authority, September 1993)

24 As long ago as 1971, a BAT document predicted: 'no further advertising within 3 years—at most within 5 years' (speaking notes entitled 'Smoking and Health Session, Chelwood, 28 May 1971: Talk 4: Likely commercial development'—Internet Ref. 1186.07 [see Note 12]). Twenty-three years later, the industry, and the Government, were still avoiding a ban on advertising, as proposed by the European Commission and by Kevin Barron MP's Private Member's Bill, by adroit use of a revision of the voluntary agreement, as is explicit in a leaked memorandum of 5 November 1993 to the Prime Minister from the Health Secretary, Mrs Virginia Bottomley

25 *The Island* (Sri Lanka). 29 October 1993

Tobacco industry tactics

Edward L Sweda Jr and **Richard A Daynard**
Tobacco Products Liability Project, School of Law, Northeastern University, Boston, Massachusetts, USA

The tobacco industry's strong-arm tactics have been used consistently over many years. These tactics include: using the industry's size, wealth, and legal resources to intimidate individuals and local governmental bodies; setting up 'front groups' to make it appear that it has more allies than it really does; spending large sums of money to frame the public debate about smoking regulations around 'rights and liberty' rather than health and portraying its tobacco company adversaries as extremists; 'investing' thousands of dollars in campaign contributions to politicians; and using financial resources to influence science. These tactics are designed to produce delay, giving the nicotine cartel more time to collect even more profits at the direct expense of millions of lives around the world.

In the field of public policy, the tobacco industry has a long and usually successful track record in influencing legislators and other decision-makers. This is especially true at the national or state level; while the industry has engaged in battles in cities and towns, its rate of success is notably poorer as they go closest to the people. Thus, the tobacco industry turns to one of its favorite strategies — pre-emption. In effect, the lesson to be learned is this: if you can't win at a particular level of government, then make that level of government irrelevant by taking away its power to act.

So, in 1994, after years of watching California communities pass and implement tough local laws requiring smoke-free public places, including restaurants, the tobacco industry poured over $18 million into a campaign to sponsor its pre-emption proposal and to collect the necessary signatures to put the proposal on the November ballot as a binding referendum. And in its efforts to obtain signatures for its effort to pre-empt local laws, Philip Morris falsely persuaded potential signers that its goal was to achieve a law to **restrict** smoking in public. California's Secretary of State, Anthony Miller, accused Philip Morris's front group — called Californians for Uniform Statewide Restrictions (CUSR) — of outright deception. CUSR made no mention of its tobacco connections. 'A great many signers have been duped, and they are furious and I don't blame them. Don't be fooled by petitions sponsored by the tobacco industry,' said Miller[1].

Once made aware of the tobacco industry's backing of Proposition 188, California voters repudiated it at the polls in November 1994, 70.5% to 29.5%.

Where they have been unsuccessful at pre-empting local authority to act, the tobacco lobby is not above acting directly to try to sway the balance on an upcoming vote by a city council. A recent example of this activity occurred in Cambridge, Massachusetts, where the city council was considering amending its existing ordinance (passed in 1987, requiring 'no-smoking' areas of at least 25% of the seating capacity in restaurants over 25 seats) to shrink any permissible smoking section to 15% of the seats. Less than a week before the scheduled vote, Philip Morris launched what the *Boston Globe* described as 'an aggressive last-minute phone bank operation' which was trying to stir up voter opposition to the ordinance[2].

Alliances with restaurant associations are nothing new for the tobacco industry. One example occurred in 1993 and 1994 in Massachusetts when Roger Donoghue worked simultaneously as a registered lobbyist at the State House for both the Massachusetts Restaurant Association and the R.J. Reynolds Tobacco Company.

A public relations effort aimed at restaurant owners across America was started in 1989 by Philip Morris. The 'Accommodation Program' was unveiled to persuade restaurants and other businesses open to the public to 'accommodate' smokers (i.e. to allow them a place to smoke in their establishment) and 'accommodate' non-smokers (i.e. to provide an area that is labeled 'no smoking,' but without any assurance, whether through separate ventilation or the physical separation of rooms, that the smoke from the smoking area would not affect those in the declared 'no smoking' area). Having published and distributed a sourcebook called, *8 Steps To Becoming An Accommodating Restaurant*, the Accommodation Program offers a 'sensible way to satisfy the preferences of non-smoking and smoking customers'. Among its tips on 'how to be an accommodating server', are: 'carry an extra pack of matches or a lighter to assist your smoking guests' and 'know where to obtain cigarettes on behalf of your guests'. Note that the sponsor, Philip Morris, is never identified in this book.

Tobacco companies have long espoused the public position that smoking is 'an adult custom'. Thus, children should simply be patient and wait until they become 18 years of age, at which time they will be sufficiently 'mature' to make a personal 'choice' as to whether or not to smoke. No mention is made of disease or addiction or anything negative about tobacco products. Rather, cigarettes are portrayed as the 'forbidden fruit' which remains ubiquitous throughout society.

The nicotine cartel has also been alarmed by the bad publicity that retailers around the US have received when they were caught illegally selling tobacco products to minors. R.J. Reynolds has launched a campaign with the national Jaycees — national Junior Chambers of Commerce — purportedly designed to discourage sales to children. In December 1990, the Tobacco Institute initiated the 'It's the Law' campaign, which featured orange and blue signs posted in stores warning that 'it's the law' that tobacco sales are prohibited to those under the age of 18. Of course, no mention is made as to **why** tobacco sales to minors should not occur. Never are any health issues raised in the industry's promotional material.

The tobacco industry has repeatedly refused to provide the public — or even its own shareholders — with evidence that would show the effectiveness or non-effectiveness of the industry-created and industry-financed campaigns against sales to minors. A glimpse of the industry's true position on this important issue can be seen in some promotional material for retailers that was disseminated by R.J. Reynolds, which designated June 1995 as 'National Awareness Month' about the problem of illegal tobacco sales to children. The R.J. Reynolds' 'Dear Retailer' letter states that 'while accessibility at retail is not the reason kids start using tobacco products, it does provide them with the opportunity to continue'. It goes on to allege: 'we also recognize the efforts of organized sting operations across the country that may have serious ramifications for retailers. These sting operations do not focus on education. The objective of these operations seems to be to make the retailer look bad rather than to work with the retailer to solve the problem.' Again, there is no mention of addiction, disease, or health in this letter to retailers.

Similarly, Philip Morris's 'PM USA NewsLine' warns retailers that 'motivated in part by a severe new federal directive, states across the country are increasingly mounting "stings" against retailers, using undercover minors to test compliance with underage sales laws. Anti-smokers are arguing for increased regulation of retailers . . .'[3]. The article goes on to cite the example of Woodridge, Illinois, where 'the village council in the town of 30,000 recently passed a new law — written by the local police — that requires sting operations on a quarterly basis, a $50 annual tobacco license fee, license suspensions for repeat violators, and fines on store owners. Since the law was implemented, 12 vendors have had their licenses suspended'. Of course, what Philip Morris omitted about Woodridge is the fact that the proportion of regular smokers in the junior high school dropped by 69%[4].

If there is not an appropriate group or entity to make an alliance with on a particular subject, the tobacco industry does the next best thing — it creates them! A prime example in the US is the National Smokers Alliance (NSA). Maintaining the guise of a spontaneous grass-roots uprising of millions of smokers outraged at the steady infringement of their God-given rights as Americans, the NSA is in reality an 'astro-turf' organization, designed to give the appearance of a legitimate expression of genuine anger at the grass roots, but created and financed by powerful outside interests. So, the NSA came into existence with the benefit of seed money from Philip Morris's public relations firm, Burson-Marsteler. It quickly claimed over a million members. The term 'member' was defined simply as someone signing his name to a form provided by signature gatherers who were paid per signature and who gave prospective 'members' free gifts, such as a key chain or lighter.

Another example of tobacco industry fabrication of allies is the United Restaurant, Hotel and Tavern Association (URHTA) of New York State which placed full-page advertisements in the *New York Times* in September 1994 to oppose the smoke-free ordinance proposed by the New York City Council. Joe Cherner of Smoke-Free Educational Services not only discovered that URHTA did not even have a telephone listing in New York City and that its supposed chapters in Queens, Brooklyn, the Bronx, and Staten Island were all defunct, but also that the URHTA representative at a City Council hearing admitted that the advertisements were, in fact, paid for by tobacco interests[5]. Similarly, in California, a group called Restaurateurs for a Sensible, Voluntary Policy (RSVP) was created by tobacco interests[6].

Not surprisingly, the 'rights' of smokers, according to the NSA, are fully consonant with the financial interests of the tobacco industry. For example, the 'right' of smokers to learn about the various ingredients in tobacco products or to bring a product liability suit against tobacco companies is not what the NSA advocates. This point was crystallized on October 28, 1994 when attorney Ronald Motley of Ness, Motley, Loadholt, Richardson & Poole cross-examined William J. Althaus, NSA chairman, at Occupational Safety and Health Administration's (OSHA) hearings on workplace smoking rules. Asked by Motley if smokers have a right to be informed about what substances are in tobacco and the impact they may have on their health, Althaus replied, 'I have no opinion on that'. When asked if he believed smoking is addictive, he replied, 'I have no idea'. While Althaus earlier had blasted the proposed OSHA regulation of smoking in the workplace as an unfair burden on NSA's members, he offered no opinion regarding the health risks of a product that will bring about the premature deaths of thousands of NSA's members[7].

An example of an NSA attempt at public education was its hiring of an airplane to tow a banner reading 'Mall St Matthews Discriminates Against Smokers', referring to a mall in Louisville, Kentucky. One might expect that a mall that truly 'discriminates' against smokers would bar them from entering the mall to shop. Instead, what got the folks at NSA agitated was that a mall in a major tobacco-growing state had the audacity to make a voluntary business decision to adopt a smoke-free policy. If one were to logically follow the reasoning behind the NSA's banner, St Matthew's Church equally 'discriminates' against smokers when it prohibits congregants from smoking during Sunday Mass.

Extremism is one of NSA's traits. The April 1995 issue of its newsletter, *NSA Voice*, quotes syndicated newspaper columnist Walter Williams, complaining about the plans of eight major airlines to ban smoking on international flights. 'Many Americans think it's good to restrict smoking and applaud the intimidation tactics by the anti-smoking lobby. We should remember that it was decent, well-meaning Germans who helped create an all-powerful government to do good things but didn't figure they were building the Trojan Horse for Adolf Hitler. Similarly, Americans are making it easy for a future tyrant.' This is NSA's response to an effort to remove a toxic pollutant from airline cabins.

Extremist language is not limited to publications that target the public at large; it can be uncovered in the industry's trade journals as well. A recent example can be found in an editorial in the April 1995 issue of *Tobacco International*. The editorial, entitled 'Blacklisting 90s Style', denounces tobacco control advocates who 'are going after the smaller, more fiscally vulnerable suppliers of tobacco flavors, papers, filters and agricultural supplies'. After predicting that the efforts of the 'antis' will fail, the editorial concludes, 'the difference is that communism is about the absence of choice, which is why it failed; smoking is about the freedom of choice, which is why it survives'[8].

Laden with money and often dissatisfied with the editorial content of newspapers and magazines, the tobacco companies have bought full-page ads, some of which appear as thinly disguised legitimate articles, in major publications across the country to send out their message on a wide variety of public policy issues affecting tobacco. A major round of such advertisements occurred shortly after a spate of negative publicity that the industry received after the Congressional hearings in the spring of 1994. R.J. Reynolds's series of ads included headlines such as 'Today It's Cigarettes. Tomorrow?', 'Smoking in a Free Society', 'Secondhand Smoke: How Much Are Non-Smokers Exposed to?' and 'Is the Government Going Too Far?' The three prongs of tobacco's propaganda are: (i) dismissing health concerns; (ii) emphasizing people's 'rights'; and (iii) bashing Government (in R.J. Reynolds's ads, the 'G' in government is **always** capitalized, thus making it bigger and more menacing).

Another means by which the tobacco industry influences the media occurred in mid-May 1995 when Philip Morris sponsored a tour of New York and Washington DC for ten Asian journalists. On the agenda for this trip were some highlights not likely to be attractions to the average visitor to these two major American cities. Topics for the journalists on the New York leg of the trip — just one month after the city's smoke-free ordinance went into effect for most restaurants — included: 'Smoking

Ban and Regulations in the US', by a speaker from the Cato Institute, a libertarian think-tank; 'Smoking Ban Impact on Chinese Restaurants', 'Smoking Ban Impact on Pubs and Restaurants' and an address by a New York City Councilman who opposed the ordinance. In Washington, the Asian journalists heard from longtime tobacco industry ally, Gary L. Huber, speaking on environmental tobacco smoke (ETS); an author from the Capital Research Centre discussing 'America, a Rising Nanny State?'; William Althaus, Chairman of NSA (who presumably did not provide transcripts of his cross-examination by Attorney Motley); and Patrick Tyson, a lawyer who represents the tobacco industry in its opposition to proposed OSHA regulations to limit smoking in the workplace.

The tobacco industry can influence public opinion in ways that are not readily apparent to the general public. For example, an editorial in the *New York Post* entitled, 'No-Smoking's Victims', berated the purported negative effects on the restaurant business inflicted by New York's smoke-free ordinance. 'This time the butt-inski brigade seems to have gone too far. The health fascists, as predicted, have actually injured a vital New York City industry,' began the editorial. What was the source of the assurance that no-smoking laws are bad for restaurant business? 'Surveys conducted independently — one by a tobacco-rights group, one by the New York Tavern and Restaurant Association — concluded that folks are staying out of eateries in large numbers'[9].

Rupert Murdoch, the Editor-in-Chief of the *New York Post*, has been a member of the Board of Directors of Philip Morris since 1989. Those who read the *Post's* vitriolic editorial that day were not apprised of that fact.

Money is in plentiful supply at tobacco industry headquarters. An article in *Business Week* details how the tobacco lobby successfully persuaded the Florida legislature to repeal a 1994 statute that makes it easier for the state of Florida to bring litigation against tobacco companies for reimbursement of Medicaid and other health benefit payments. The article, entitled, 'Full-Flavored, Unfiltered Statehouse Shenanigans', described the 'Tobacco Team' — the two dozen lobbyists who descended on the Florida legislature in Tallahassee. 'The industry relied on its traditional strengths: money, power, and influence. The combination worked once again — proof that tobacco makers are far from vanquished by negative public opinion and antismoking legislation.' Governor Lawton Chiles has promised to veto the repeal of the statute. The article concludes: 'polls indicate two-thirds of Floridians favor his law, and he'll work to lure enough Democratic legislators to avoid an override. But Team Tobacco has staying power. Public opinion is against it. Yet money, and legal acumen, often talk louder than voters[10].'

An example of the tobacco industry's proclivity to bully small municipalities occurred in late 1994 in the town of Puyallup,

Washington. The Puyallup City Council passed an ordinance on August 1 to require all restaurants in that city of 27,000 to be smoke-free as of January 1, 1995. However, on December 19, less than two weeks before the new law was to take effect, the council voted 6 to 1 to reverse itself and repeal the ordinance. What had happened in the intervening months that had such a profound effect on the city councillors?

On November 29, nine restaurants in Puyallup filed a civil rights suit to challenge the ordinance. Among the allegations contained in the complaint filed by the plaintiffs was the assertion that the ordinance was pre-empted by state law because the Washington Clean Indoor Air Act, set forth at RCW 70.160, permitted smoking sections in restaurants. The plaintiffs also imaginatively alleged that the city had unlawfully and substantially deprived plaintiffs' rights guaranteed by the US Constitution including, but not limited to, violating the 'takings' clause (which requires the Government to pay compensation for private property which it seizes) of the Fifth Amendment.

The lawsuit was financed by the R.J. Reynolds Tobacco Co. Rather than expend the funds necessary to fight the lawsuit in court, the City Council backed down and decided to repeal the ordinance before the public had any opportunity to benefit from it. Tobacco money had once again prevailed over the public health.

According to *Can't Kick the Habit . . . The Tobacco Industry & Washington*, a lengthy study unveiled in March 1995 by Common Cause, a citizens' lobbying group, 'twelve tobacco industry companies and lobbying groups, along with their executives, gave a total of $16,738,872 in political action committee (PAC) and soft money contributions during the past decade — a decade in which increasing public scrutiny of the health effects of smoking and tobacco use resulted in relatively little congressional action on anti-tobacco legislation'. Common Cause President, Ann McBride, said that the 'tobacco lobby's use of political contributions is a classic example of the influence-money scandal at work in Washington. Members of Congress are as addicted to large campaign contributions as smokers are to nicotine.' The breakdown was as follows: Philip Morris $5,083,557; R.J. Reynolds $4,879,975; US Tobacco $2,882,438; and Tobacco Institute $1,618,979.

The recipients of the campaign contribution money were not chosen at random. For example, in the spring of 1994, legislation to ban smoking in most public buildings was approved by the House Subcommittee on Health and the Environment and sent along to the full Energy and Commerce Committee. The full committee postponed scheduled mark-ups on that bill (H.R. 3434) and never took final action on it. Members of the 103rd Congress who served on the Energy and Commerce Committee received $860,658 from tobacco industry PACs during the decade 1985–1994 (an average of $19,560 each). The average member of

Congress over that same time span received $9,409 from tobacco PACs, less than half of the amount received by committee members[11].

Glantz and Begay have documented the significant influence of tobacco industry campaign contributions on state lawmakers in California, independent of their constituents' support for tobacco control[12].

Tobacco companies are equally virulent in their use of the judicial system to intimidate those who would criticize or regulate them. While the combined resources of scientists, NGOs, the media, and local and national governments obviously far exceed the wealth of even the tobacco industry, the industry is able to threaten and deter (though only rarely to defeat) individuals and entities in each of these categories through a 'divide and conquer' strategy.

Beginning in 1953, the industry adopted 'a holding strategy'[13], consisting of:

- creating doubt about the health charge without actually denying it.
- advocating the public's right to smoke, without actually urging them to take up the practice.
- encouraging objective scientific research as the only way to resolve the question of health hazard.

As for individual scientists who had reached troublesome findings, Philip Morris in 1981 proposed 'attacking researchers themselves, where vulnerable'[14]. Current and former employees and contractors are held on a tight leash: thus, R.J. Reynolds Tobacco Co. obtained an injunction to keep a former scientist from discussing work done for the company to determine how smoking causes emphysema[15], while Council for Tobacco Research agents threatened a major recipient of research funds that publishing his result—that inhaling smoke does cause cancer in laboratory animals—would end their relationship. When he published anyway, his funding was indeed cut off, and his efforts to publicize his results were surreptitiously undermined[16].

Avoiding Faustian bargains with the tobacco industry does not protect scientists from harassment and intimidation, however. Dr Irving Selikoff's data for his pathbreaking studies on the relationship between asbestos exposure, smoking, and lung cancer were subpoenaed by the tobacco industry[17], as were the records of the process leading up to the various Surgeon General's reports on smoking and health[18], as were the data and other records of the researchers who concluded that the 'Joe Camel' advertising campaign appealed to children and teenagers[19].

Even reporting studies done by others can be hazardous, if the tobacco industry is displeased. In 1987 the Dutch Foundation on Smoking and Health (StiVoRo) dared to state, as part of a public education campaign, that passive smoking badly affects one's health. The joint tobacco manufacturers quickly sued, accusing StiVoRo of 'misleading the public'. The court sided with StiVoRo, and the tobacco companies finally withdrew their claims and agreed to pay legal costs[20]. But, for 42 months, StiVoRo was distracted from its tobacco control efforts by having to fight this rearguard action. News media have had the same experience: Philip Morris filed a $10 billion lawsuit against the American Broadcasting Company and two of its journalists for daring to suggest that the industry 'spiked' cigarettes with nicotine[21].

It is perhaps not surprising that the industry feels free to sue local governments like Puyallup, Washington (discussed above), Province-town, Massachusetts (unsuccessful industry effort to overturn ban on cigarette vending machines), or even New York City (successful 'pre-emption' attack on ban on taxicab-top cigarette advertising)[22]. But the industry has also taken on the US Environmental Protection Agency (for daring to conclude that environmental tobacco smoke causes lung cancer) and the Canadian Government (for presuming to have the constitutional power to ban cigarette advertising)[23]. Presently, it is threatening governments throughout the world with the preposterous legal claim that label regulations infringe the companies' trademark rights, in violation of international conventions.

The point of these tactics — whether political, public relations, or legal — is not to win. The tobacco executives know that, at least in developed countries, they are fighting a losing battle. But the tactics do succeed in distracting and intimidating tobacco control forces, and delaying (and occasionally reversing) tobacco control gains. And every year of delay means billions of dollars in profits, albeit at the cost of millions of lives.

Acknowledgements

The authors wish to thank Ann B. Toback for her assistance in preparing this article.

References

1 *San Francisco Chronicle* April 18, 1994
2 Philips F. Tobacco firms court Cambridge smokers. *Boston Globe*, May 6, 1995, pp 13, 20; and Paige C. Tobacco giant's campaign calls on Cambridge residents. *Boston Herald* May 6, 1995, p 7
3 Legislation may threaten retail sales. *PM USA NewsLine* (Retailer Edn) Winter 1995: p 1
4 DiFranza JR. Active enforcement of minors' access: a moral and ethical imperative. *Tobacco Control* 1995; 4: 5
5 Smith L. Big Apple breathes easy. *Tobacco Control* 1995; 4: 15–17

6   Glantz SA, Smith LRA. The effect of ordinances requiring smoke-free restaurants on restaurant sales. *Am J Public Health* 1994; **84**: 1081–5

7   National Smokers Alliance Chairman cross-examined by Castano Litigator at OSHA Indoor Air Quality Hearing. *Tobacco Products Litigation Reporter* 1994; **9** (5): 1.88, 1.89

8   *Tobacco International* April 1995: p 3

9   No-smoking's victims. *New York Post* May 18, 1995: p 22

10 Mallory M. Full-flavored, unfiltered Statehouse shenanigans. *Business Week* May 22, 1995: p 52

11 Can't kick the habit. *Common Cause* media release. March 24, 1995. This study does not address the tobacco industry's contributions to officials at the state or local level

12 Glantz SA, Begay NE. Tobacco industry campaign contributions are affecting tobacco control policymaking in California. *JAMA* 1994; **272**: 1176–82

13 Memorandum to Horace R. Kornegay from Fred Panzer, May 1, 1972. Exh. P-1 105, Cipollone vs Liggett Group, Inc., reprinted in *Tobacco Products Litigation Reporter* 1988; **3** (4): 3.3 68–3.370

14 Memorandum to H. Cullman/J.C. Bowling from J.J. Morgan, March 24. 1981, Exh. P-2745, Cipollone vs Liggett Group, Inc., reprinted in *Tobacco Products Litigation Reporter* 1988; &B3 (5): 3.423

15 R.J. Reynolds Tobacco Co. vs Colluci, 8.2 TPLR 2.225 (N.C. Super. Ct. 1993)

16 Confidential memorandum to 'Henry-Tom' from Leonard Zahn, April 22, 1974, Exh. P-1205A, Cipollone vs Liggett Group, Inc., reprinted in *Tobacco Products Litigation Reporter* 1988; **3** (5): 3.416–3.417

17 Mt Sinai School of Medicine vs American Tobacco Co., 866 F.2d 552 (2d Cir. 1989)

18 Cipollone vs Liggett Group, Inc., 2.7 TPLR 2.119 (US Ct. App., 4th Cir. 1987)

19 DiFranza JR. If the science is irrefutable, attack the scientist. *Tobacco Control* 1992; **1**: 237–8

20 DeJong R. A defeat for the tobacco industry. *World Smoking Health* 1992; **17**: 23

21 Skolnick AA. Burning mad tobacco firms turn up heat on major news media. *Newsletter of the National Association of Screenwriters* 1994; **42**: 1–5

22 Take Five Vending Co. vs Provincetown, 415 Mass. 741, 615 NE 2d 576 (1993); Vango Media vs City of New York, 829 F. Supp. 572 (SDNY 1993)

23 Flue-Cured Tobacco Cooperative Stabilization Corp. vs EPA, 857 F. Supp. 1137 (MDNC 1994); Ronson J, Cunningham R. Fighting for health: the Canadian tobacco advertising case. *World Smoking Health* 1992; **17**: 24–5

Product modification

Robert E Waller* and **Peter Froggatt**[†]

Former *Scientific Secretary and [†]Chairman, Independent Scientific Committee on Smoking and Health, UK

For more than 20 years there has been a coherent programme of product modification in the UK, involving the introduction of low tar brands of cigarettes and the gradual reduction in average tar yields over the whole range of manufactured cigarettes. The sales-weighted average tar yield has declined from 20.8 mg/cigarette in 1972 to 11.0 mg/cigarette in 1993. To some extent potential benefits to established smokers have been offset by their tendency to 'compensate' for reduced nicotine yields. Investigating such aspects has formed one part of a wide-ranging research programme to monitor effects of modified products on health. Collectively the studies show benefits in terms of smoke intake and health outcome related to reduced tar cigarettes, but the success achieved in reducing average tar yields and narrowing the range has limited opportunities to detect differential effects.

Following the findings in the early 1950s of the strong association between cigarette smoking and lung cancer[1-7], evidence soon accumulated linking smoking with other adverse effects[8]. Government and the health authorities, though quickly accepting the major findings[9], responded warily — and to many, inadequately — mainly through pressure on the industry to curtail its more extravagant marketing practices, through public awareness campaigns, and through advising smokers to stop and others not to start. The determinants and gradual development of policies have been described in detail elsewhere [10]. Despite these moves and accumulating medical evidence, total cigarette smoking, especially by women, rose inexorably[11] and by the early 1970s it was clear that more vigorous policies were required. These were increasingly focused on the toxicity of tobacco components and on product regulation, and a key move was to establish, in 1973, the Independent Scientific Committee on Smoking and Health (ISCSH) to advise Health Ministers and, where appropriate, the tobacco companies on the scientific aspects of matters concerning smoking and health[12]. Until its replacement (in 1994 — see 'TPRT' below) the Committee has been at the centre of helping to formulate national smoking and health policies framed in the interests of the public health.

Its creation was timely. Throughout the 1950s and 1960s there were numerous developments in the US and Europe towards 'less harmful'

Address for correspondence: Mr Robert E Waller, Department of Health, Wellington House, 133–155 Waterloo Road, London SE1 8UG, UK

©The British Council 1996

cigarettes[13]. These involved tobacco technology — such as using some reconstituted tobacco sheet — but importantly also the introduction of filters, an outstanding marketing success driven by commercial rather than health considerations since (in the UK) excise duty was then levied on the tobacco content of cigarettes, enabling filter-tips to be sold more cheaply. Thus, between 1956 and 1970, consumption of cigarette tobacco declined by 9.6% but cigarettes sold increased by 28.5% by which time 4 in every 5 cigarettes were tipped[11]. Some, however, were designed to reduce 'tar', the particulate phase of cigarette smoke then held responsible for the carcinogenic activity[14]. These developments did not amount to a coherent, monitored policy, and it was the initial task of ISCSH to devise one. This required Government resolve and industry cooperation, clearly neither initially assured, and the determinants and developments of these have been fully described by one of us[10]. It is sufficient to say here that the programme designed by ISCSH, agreed by the tobacco industry, and negotiated by Government with the Tobacco Advisory Council (TAC) as part of a series of so-called 'voluntary agreements' in 1973, 1977, 1980 and 1984 is known as the 'product modification programme'. No country then, or since, has developed such a regulatory system, and it is described in detail in the ISCSH Fourth Report[12].

Tobacco 'substitutes' and 'additives'

The first step in the programme was a radical one: the feasibility and advantages of introducing synthetic tobacco substitutes to cigarettes to replace some of the natural tobacco. This required extensive testing of the toxicity of the substances themselves, in various mixtures with tobacco, and of the resultant smoke; and the formulation of testing guidelines for additives generally[15]. The original substitutes tested were 'New Smoking Material' (NSM) and Cytrel, each based on modified cellulose. They were submitted to ISCSH in 1973 but, because of the thoroughness of the test procedures, were not cleared for marketing until April 1977. On 1 July that year, 11 brands (and in a fortnight a twelfth) were launched each containing 25% 'substitute' and 75% natural tobacco. Consumer uptake was initially satisfactory but rapidly fell off for a variety of reasons; sales were soon negligible and the brands were withdrawn with much financial loss to the companies involved[16]. The invaluable toxicological testing expertise gained by the ISCSH was recognised by vesting the responsibility for approving all additives in the Committee, as part of the Voluntary Agreement of 1977, rather than in the Customs and Excise as previously, an authority which ISCSH has used judiciously but

Table 1 Definition of tar bands

From 1972	Tar yield, mg/cigarette
Low	10 or less
Low to middle	11–16
Middle	17–22
Middle to high	23–28
High	29 or more*
From 1985	
Low	under 10
Low to middle	10 but less than 15
Middle	15 but less than 18
High	18 and above

*The highest quoted yield in 1972 was 38 mg. This band disappeared in 1980. The banding system was phased out during 1992, when actual yields of tar and nicotine were required to be printed on packets. From 31 December 1992, an absolute upper limit of 15 mg tar was imposed by regulation, and the limit is due to fall to 12 mg from 31 December 1997.

constructively as part of its later policies to make lower-yield cigarettes more acceptable to recalcitrant smokers.

Tar reduction

The failure of the 'substitutes' sounded a knell for radicalism in product modification; thereafter, the ISCSH and the tobacco industry were forced to a strategy of gradualism, reducing tobacco yields by such means as effective filters, increasing the porosity of cigarette papers, introducing ventilation holes near the tip of the cigarette, and ingenuities in tobacco chemistry and blending. Though aimed primarily at 'tar', they also reduced the yields of nicotine and of some gaseous components, though not necessarily *pro rata*[12], so that any harmful effects of non-tar components would also be reduced *pari passu*. Since July 1972, monitoring of (machine) yields of 'tar' and nicotine (and later of carbon monoxide) has been carried out by the Laboratory of the Government Chemist (LGC) through biannual surveys showing manufacturers' brands in rank order of tar yield within various tar-delimited 'bands' (Table 1), published by the Department of Health, over much of the time in leaflet and poster form for public information.

This policy of gradualism was based on two assumptions. First, that the important noxious materials — especially the carcinogenic ones — are in the tobacco tar and/or other products of combustion with a dose response relationship between the yields and smoking-related diseases without a significant threshold of safety. Evidence with respect to lung cancer at least favours this. In fact, since the programme also reduces nicotine and (some) gases, for it to be justifiable the noxa need not be in the 'tar' fraction. Second, that the programme is not such as to prompt significant 'consumer-resistance', i.e. through smoking more cigarettes; by switching to a stronger brand; or by 'over-smoking' a cigarette — longer and more frequent puffs, shorter butts, deeper pulls, etc., any of which would increase the smoker's tar exposure. The ISCSH consistently advised people not to smoke but could have little to say on commercial measures to combat the numbers of cigarettes smoked (e.g. advertising, tobacco tax) but it acted in two ways to reduce the toxicity of products available to smokers.

First, to encourage health-conscious but recalcitrant smokers, new products were introduced in the low tar band (<10 mg/cigarette) and smokers were encouraged by advice and selective advertising to switch to them: by February 1986, 33 of 138 brands in the LGC survey list were low tar as against only 13 of 121 in 1976[11]. This had an early, but later a less marked, success: the low tar brand market, less than 1% in 1974 rose steadily but plateaued around 15% in the 1980s. However, as yields of all products fall further to comply with new regulations, the market share in the low-tar range is tending to increase again.

Second, the yields of non-low-tar brands have been gradually lowered and the strong brand loyalty of most smokers has ensured very little switching to higher-yield brands. For monitoring, sales-weighted average tar yields (SWAT) were calculated across all tar bands pooled for each survey period using LGC data and industry figures for brand market share, with similar indices for nicotine and later carbon monoxide (Fig. 1).

Targets for SWAT were set in successive voluntary agreements based on proportionate rather than absolute reductions, and the 1980 Agreement specified a SWAT target of 15 mg/cigarette by the end of 1983 — which was completely met — and of 'approximately' 13 mg/cigarette by the end of 1987[17] — which was nearly met. This policy was fortified by re-defining tar bands (Table 1), by restricting tar yields of new brands to 13 mg[17] and setting progressively reducing tar limits for existing brands[12]. This latter method has become the major thrust of product modifications in the 1990s as regulatory controls implementing EU Directives replace, in the UK, the voluntary agreements and bring the other EU countries under regulation based on this cornerstone of UK practice. Currently, there is an upper limit of brand tar yield of 15 mg/cigarette, set to become 12 mg by the end of 1997, though with some derogation for one member state. The UK is among the leaders with a SWAT now of only some 11 mg/cigarette (Fig. 1). In retrospect, the operational success of the product modification programme owes more to the gradual decrease in tar yields of popular mid-tar brands and consumer brand loyalty than to significant and deliberate switching by

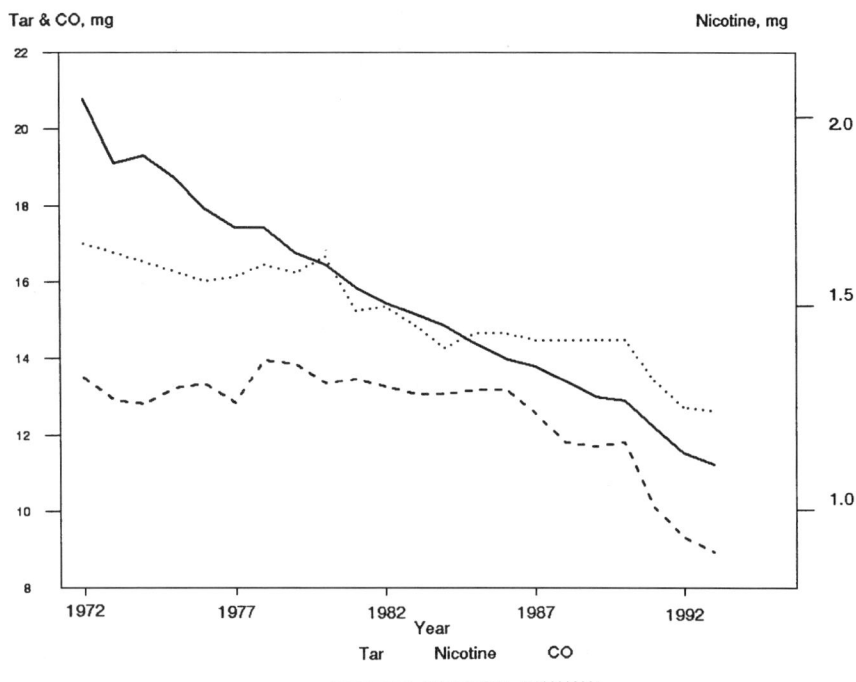

Tar & CO, mg   Nicotine, mg

Fig. 1 Trends in sales–weighted–average yields of tar, nicotine and carbon monoxide from UK cigarettes since 1972, mg per cigarette. Calendar year averages based on a combination of data from the Laboratory of the Government Chemist, the Tobacco Manufacturers' Association and the ICRF Health Behaviour Unit.

smokers into low-tar brands. In consequence, the range of tar yields has contracted with brands, originally high-tar, having fallen most (Fig. 2). This is welcome to the public health but has had an inconvenient result: reduction in brand tar yield variance has made epidemiological studies of the effect of tar-yield on smoking-related diseases increasingly difficult as the ISCSH sponsored research proceeded (see 'TPRT' below).

Nicotine yields and 'compensatory smoking'

We have mentioned that the programme has depended *inter alia* on ensuring, as far as possible, that cigarettes with reduced yields are not 'over-smoked' otherwise uptake of 'tar' by the individual smoker could remain little changed, i.e. he (or she) will 'compensate' for the lower yields.

Such 'compensatory smoking' is motivated mainly, though not exclusively, by the need of individuals permanently or intermittently to restore their nicotine uptake per cigarette to their customary level without switching brands[18]. Until 1972, brand yields of nicotine decreased reasonably *pro rata* with tar, since steps to reduce one also reduced the other. Since then, commercial imperatives (retaining brand market share)

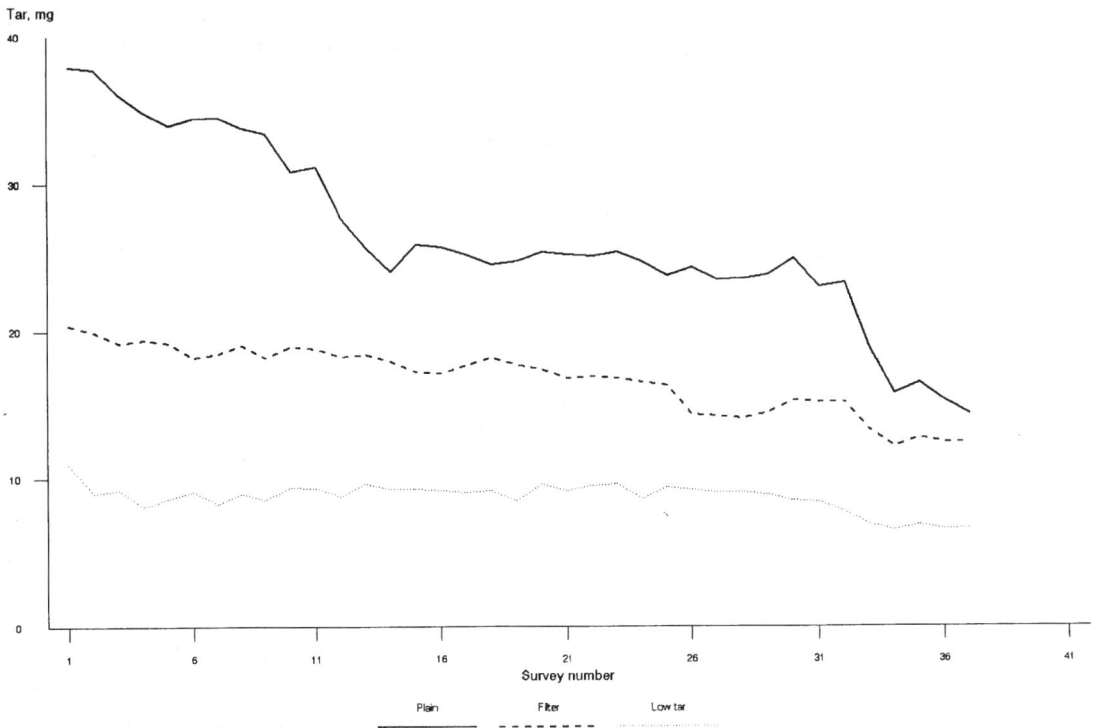

Fig. 2 Trends in tar yields for three representative brands of cigarettes monitored continuously from Survey 1 (July–December 1972) to Survey 37 (November 1993–April 1994).

have forced manufacturers to maintain nicotine yields as 'tar' has declined under the product modification programme. This was cautiously tolerated by the ISCSH who saw the use of consumer-optimum levels of nicotine (1.2–1.3 mg/cigarette in UK), which the evidence then suggested was not harmful to health, as a means of preserving brand loyalty as (harmful) tar was progressively reduced. Thus, between 1975 and 1987, sales-weighted average nicotine yields remained relatively unchanged while SWAT fell by 23%. Low nicotine brands, and the proportion of smokers smoking them, both increased — respectively from 23 to 37, and from 5% to 16%[11]. Clearly, there are technological limits to this approach and it also raises moral, philosophical, and political issues concerning using an habituating drug in this way, especially in the young and new smoker. It also supposes that nicotine in these doses is not harmful — a challenged assumption[19,20]. Nevertheless, ISCSH saw it as making a virtue out of a practical necessity, while also recommending future falls in sales-weighted average nicotine[12], which are now taking place. While a revised standard analytical method accounted for part of the decline around 1991, there is now a clear downward trend in nicotine yields, in line with the enforced reduction in tar yields (Fig. 1).

This programme could be compromised by 'compensatory smoking'. The routine smoked-tobacco compounds' determinations are made on smoking machines using internationally agreed puff parameters[21] which, if varied, may change the absolute readings but not the rank order of brands for each component[12]. Nevertheless, the degree of 'compensation', i.e. individual uptake compared to machine-yield, is important. Biochemical markers in blood, urine or saliva, of which the nicotine metabolite cotinine is the most frequently used, can serve as measures of nicotine uptake, and proxies of uptake of other components and studies among smokers of different products[22] and of those switching from higher to lower yielding ones[23], generally show partial, but not complete, 'compensation'. To an extent 'compensation', therefore, reduces machine-yield-predicted advantages of lower-yielding products, but since under the programme tar yields have been allowed to fall appreciably more than nicotine yields, average tar uptake by individuals is still reduced. Furthermore, only exceptionally, if at all, could 'compensation' lead to uptakes even approaching machine-yields of 30 years ago (in 1965, SWAT was 31.5 mg/cigarette and SWAN 2.08 mg/cigarette[11]), so that the product modification has led to a significant reduction in 'tar' uptake per cigarette in nearly all smokers. More detailed information on the extent to which smokers compensate for reduced yields in modern cigarettes is now emerging from the TPRT research programme (see below).

Carbon monoxide and other smoke components

Carbon monoxide yields have been monitored routinely since 1976. The view of the ISCSH since its Third Report is that yields should be reduced on health grounds[17], but the reductions have not been as marked as those for tar (Fig. 1). Straightforward filtration has little effect on the gaseous components: only with ventilation techniques, as used in low-tar brands, are vapour-phase as well as particulate fractions reduced. This has meant that other gaseous components, possibly toxic, which would have been reduced *pari passu* with carbon monoxide, remain largely unchanged. This is undesirable since a basic empiric advantage of the product modification programme was that reductions in major and monitored particulate and gaseous phase components would be accompanied by reduction in other (recognised or unrecognised), possibly harmful, substances. A number of additional analytes which in higher concentrations in animals were known to be harmful were therefore studied. Brand yields from the LGC survey for October 1982–March 1983 were measured for total aldehydes, nitric oxide, hydrogen cyanide, acrolein and formaldehyde[12], and repeated for selected brands 3 years later[12], with phenols and PAHs subsequently added[24]. The mostly high positive inter-correlations[12] indicated justification for our empiricism and a policy of selective reduction was therefore not required. Nitric oxide was an exception but only in some continental and American brands which have relatively high nitrate contents[12,24].

Innovative products

In an effort to reduce the levels of harmful pyrolysis products and to produce less sidestream smoke, there have been developments of products that 'heat rather than burn tobacco'. One design, that has been the subject of extensive toxicological testing[25] comprises a carbon heat source, an aluminium capsule, spray-dried tobacco, glycerol, flavour, a tobacco-paper filter, a polypropylene filter and several sections of paper. Externally, the product is similar to a conventional cigarette and the smoker receives a glycerol-based aerosol carrying the nicotine and flavours from the tobacco, together with carbon monoxide and other vapour components. There have also been proposals to use electric heaters rather than carbon in such devices[26], but to date none of these products has been marketed successfully. Clearly such developments would radically change the concept of product modification and their impact in relation to public health would need careful scrutiny.

Product modification and smoking-related diseases

However valid the *a priori* case for the low-tar programme, its ultimate justification must depend on whether or not it contributes significantly to reducing the incidence of smoking-related diseases. We have argued that the programme's role in reducing lung cancer mortality, especially in younger age groups (who have not been exposed to high tar products in their shorter smoking history), has been established[12,27,28]. This is now supported by recent national data[29]. These show deaths from lung cancer now declining at all ages among men and under 65 years among women (Table 2), the trends being best interpretable as cohort effects with men born in the early 1900s — who reached smoking age at or after World War I, and women born in the 1920s — who reached smoking age at or after World War II, having the highest death rates. This decline in mortality has occurred more than expected on the basis of cigarette consumption alone, indicating that product modification has played a

Table 2 Mortality rate per million in Britain from lung cancer by age, sex and calendar year

	Males										
	30–34	35–39	40–44	45–49	50–54	55–59	60–64	65–69	70–74	75–79	80–84
1951–55	37	102	251	591	1244	2024	2564	2909	2568	2026	1413
1956–60	35	95	256	599	1262	2326	3368	3944	3861	3289	2221
1961–65	34	95	229	575	1241	2319	3716	4882	4974	4494	3367
1966–70	26	77	225	540	1170	2226	3719	5304	6213	5933	4525
1971–75	23	59	180	510	1081	2090	3554	5195	6825	7243	6058
1976–80	17	54	139	401	1009	1908	3346	4977	6692	7987	7638
1981–85	13	42	120	322	780	1731	3021	4574	6336	7753	8395
1986–90	8	34	104	276	600	1350	2691	4129	5850	7135	7975
1991–92	9	33	91	250	612	1135	2241	3936	5312	6542	7518

	Females										
	30–34	35–39	40–44	45–49	50–54	55–59	60–64	65–69	70–74	75–79	80–84
1951–55	15	28	52	89	139	207	286	352	391	440	398
1956–60	15	31	63	105	171	243	331	387	454	496	459
1961–65	11	32	71	140	219	308	424	518	548	580	564
1966–70	11	31	82	164	286	401	512	653	729	740	671
1971–75	8	28	70	187	339	504	678	807	880	901	868
1976–80	7	27	65	164	374	583	869	1033	1112	1134	1060
1981–85	7	25	61	147	315	650	992	1313	1450	1462	1360
1986–90	6	21	63	141	276	583	1131	1496	1757	1769	1663
1991–92	4	17	62	147	289	499	1019	1608	1891	1976	1827

role in men under 60 beginning after 1965 and now emerging in young women[29].

A major problem in evaluating benefits of tar reduction in any more quantitative sense is that the risks of lung cancer in individuals are liable to be related to their whole histories of smoking, extending back to the high yielding products of much earlier decades, and yields of those smoked more recently provide little guide to overall exposures. There have, over the same period, also been favourable changes in some other factors of possible relevance to lung cancer risks, such as exposure to coal smoke. An increasing risk of lung cancer with both number of cigarettes smoked per day and tar yields has been reported from a prospective study in the US[30] and the authors considered that reductions in lung cancer risks were to be anticipated among smokers whose lifetime habits embraced only low-tar cigarettes. Support for this has come also from a case-control study[31] in which a significant trend in lung cancer risk in relation to tar yield was demonstrated.

Of the other 'smoking-related' diseases, of which the International Agency for Research on Cancer (IARC) lists some 30 within ICD numbers[32], the programme has probably been beneficial in chronic obstructive airway disease[27] but its role with respect to the others, including ischaemic heart disease, has not been unequivocally established.

Future studies, including several on-going ones sponsored by the Tobacco Products Research Trust (see below), should elucidate some of these.

The product modification programme has also been beneficial in other ways: the reduction in the toxicity of cigarettes and the continued publication of their tar yields have reinforced the hazards of smoking, thereby encouraging some people to stop smoking as well as switching to lower tar brands, themselves less harmful and often a first step to complete cessation.

At the end of 1991, with the new regulatory controls on tar yields being introduced, the ISCSH was disbanded, to be followed by the establishment, in 1994, of the Scientific Committee on Tobacco and Health, with a wider remit.

The Tobacco Products Research Trust (TPRT)

The ISCSH early recognised that the auditing of the product modification programme must include research to assess its effect on the health of smokers. This would require a coherent, ISCSH-planned, research programme; eclectic research findings from the world literature would be inadequate. Under the Voluntary Agreements of 1980 and 1984 sums of up to £1m p.a. during 1981–1987 were made available by the tobacco industry through the Tobacco Advisory Council (TAC) for 'independent monitoring research into the effect on the health of smokers of modifications of tobacco products'. The ISCSH considered it advisable to establish a charitable Trust to administer these funds and the TPRT was registered with the Charity Commissioners in 1982. Applications were sought through advertisements in the medical and national press, and all grant and contract submissions were considered by ISCSH using referee systems and 'best practice', those approved being recommended to the Trust for funding. In this way an extensive programme of relevant research, latterly wider than direct epidemiological 'intervention' studies aimed to differentiate between effects of different types of products, which were operationally and technically difficult, was compiled. The Trust effectively terminated on 31 May 1995 with 36 projects completed, many large-scale fully funded, over 100 publications in scientific journals with others in preparation and over £8m committed. Three international symposia were also organised[18,33,34], the last two jointly with the Department of Health. It appears likely that the product modification programme will be further vindicated by the results of some of these studies, including new information in relation to ischaemic heart disease[35]. The latter study also investigated the effect of compensatory smoking on the uptake of smoke components by smokers of products in different tar bands, reporting that the mean plasma cotinine level was 19% higher in the medium-tar as compared with the low-tar group, not as great a difference as the 52% difference in mean yields of nicotine, but still representing a helpful reduction in uptake for low-tar products.

Detailed analyses of the uptake of both nicotine and carbon monoxide have also been reported recently from the 'tar reduction study' carried out under the TPRT programme[36]. Overall compensation for carbon monoxide was 65.4% and for nicotine 78.8%, the lower value for carbon monoxide reflecting the fact that the proportionate reduction in the yield of low tar to high tar cigarettes is greater for carbon monoxide than for nicotine. A full description of the Trust and its sponsored research will be published shortly[37]: some of the earlier studies have already been reviewed[12].

Conclusion

Since the early 1970s, product modification has formed part of the overall strategy to reduce the impact of smoking on public health. There has been a substantial reduction in the prevalence of smoking among adults, resulting from cessation activities[38] and trends in a number of smoking-related diseases are becoming more favourable[29]. The specific role of product modification is difficult to separate from that of changes in prevalence, but much evidence has accumulated to show that smoke intake has been reduced, and consequent reductions in adverse effects are to be anticipated. The prime message must at all times be not to smoke, but for the dependent adult smoker who fails to heed such advice there is no longer any access to strong high-yielding products, and, with current policies forcing tar yields and effectively nicotine yields down even further there is the prospect too that young people who may still experiment with smoking at an early age will be less likely to become addicted and to continue the habit. Providing that governments or smokers do not come to regard reductions in tar yields as substitutes for the avoidance of cigarettes, the further reduction, to 12 mg/cigarette in the regulatory upper limit, will help to reduce the number of premature deaths from tobacco[35].

Acknowledgements

The views expressed in this article are the personal views of the authors and they do not necessarily reflect those of other members of the former

Independent Scientific Committee on Smoking and Health, or of the Department of Health, or of other organisations referred to.

All the analytical work referred to here was undertaken by the Laboratory of the Government Chemist (LGC) and we would like to thank Geoffrey Phillips and Keith Darrall in particular for supplying data. The Tobacco Manufacturers' Association provided information on sales-weighted averages, based on LGC analyses, and we would also like to thank Martin Jarvis of the ICRF Health Behaviour Unit for further contributions on this topic. The product modification programme owes much of its success to the guidance provided by members of the Independent Scientific Committee on Smoking and Health and we are indebted to the Trustees of the Tobacco Products Research Trust and to the Scientific Liaison Officer, Cheryl Swann, for their contributions on research aspects.

References

1   Schrek R, Baker A, Ballard GP, Dolgoff S. Tobacco smoking as an etiologic factor in disease. 1. Cancer. *Cancer Res* 1950; **10**: 49–58

2   Mills CA, Porter MM. Tobacco smoking habits and cancer of the mouth and respiratory system. *Cancer Res* 1950; **10**: 539–42

3   Levin ML, Goldstein H, Gerhardt PR. Cancer and tobacco smoking. *JAMA* 1950; **143**: 336–8

4   Wynder EL, Graham EA. Tobacco smoking as a possible etiologic factor in bronchogenic carcinoma. A study of six hundred and eighty four proved cases. *JAMA* 1950; **143**: 329–36

5   Doll R, Hill AB. Smoking and carcinoma of the lung: preliminary report. *BMJ* 1950; **2**: 739–48

6   McConnell RR, Gordon KCT, Jones T. Occupational and personal factors in the aetiology of carcinoma of the lung. *Lancet* 1952; **2**: 651–6

7   Doll R, Hill AB. A study of the aetiology of cancer of the lung. *BMJ* 1952; **2**: 1271–86

8   Royal College of Physicians of London. *Smoking and Health*. London: Pitman Medical, 1962

9   Hansard HC, 1953–4, vol 523, col 173-4W

10 Froggatt P. Determinants of policy on smoking and health. *Int J Epidemiol* 1989; **18**: 1–9.

11 Wald N, Kiryluk S, Darby S, Doll R, Pike M, Peto R. eds. *UK Smoking Statistics*. Oxford: Oxford University Press, 1988

12 Independent Scientific Committee on Smoking and Health. Fourth Report. London: HMSO, 1988

13 National Cancer Institute. *Toward a less harmful cigarette*. Monograph 28. Bethesda MD: National Cancer Institute, 1968

14 Wynder EL, Hoffmann D. *Tobacco and Tobacco Smoke*. New York: Academic Press, 1967

15 Independent Scientific Committee on Smoking and Health. First report. London: HMSO: 1975

16 Van Rossum R. The great substitute disaster. *The Grocer*; 16 September 1978

17 Independent Scientific Committee on Smoking and Health. Third Report. London: HMSO: 1983

18 Wald N, Froggatt P. eds. *Nicotine, Smoking and the Low Tar Programme*. Oxford: Oxford University Press, 1989: Section III, pp 85–236

19 Hoffmann D. Nicotine, a tobacco-specific precursor for carcinogenesis. In: Wald N, Froggatt P. eds. *Nicotine, Smoking and the Low Tar Programme*. Oxford: Oxford University Press 1989: pp 24–40

20 Editorial. Nicotine use after the year 2000. *Lancet* 1991; **337**: 1191–2

21 Johnson JC. The development of machine smoking parameters for the measurement of cigarette tar yield in the United Kingdom. *J Assoc Off Anal Chem* 1986; **69**: 598–600

22 Wald NJ, Boreham J, Bailey A. Relative intakes of tar, nicotine and carbon monoxide from cigarettes of different yields. *Thorax* 1984; **39**: 361–4

23 Benowitz NL, Jacob P. Nicotine and carbon monoxide intake from high and low yield cigarettes. *Clin Pharmacol Ther* 1984; **36**: 265–9

24 Phillips GF, Waller RE. Yields of tar and other smoke components from UK cigarettes. *Food Chem Toxicol* 1991; **29**: 469–74

25 RJ Reynolds Tobacco Company. *Chemical and biological studies on new cigarette prototypes that heat instead of burn tobacco.* Winston-Salem NC: RJ Reynolds Tobacco Company, 1988

26 Davis RM, Slade J. Back to the future—with electrically powered cigarettes. *Tobacco Control* 1993; **2**: 11–12

27 Darby SC, Doll R, Stratton IM. Trends in mortality from smoking related diseases in England and Wales. In: Wald N, Froggatt P. eds. *Nicotine, Smoking and the Low Tar Programme.* Oxford: Oxford University Press, 1989: pp 70–82

28 Froggatt P, Wald N. The role of nicotine in the tar reduction programme. In: Wald N, Froggatt P. eds. *Nicotine, Smoking and the Low Tar Programme.* Oxford: Oxford University Press, 1989: pp 229–35

29 Doll R, Darby S, Whitley E. Trends in smoking related diseases. In: Charlton J, Murphy M. eds. *The Health of Adult Britain, 1841–1991.* Decennial Supplement, Office of Population Censuses and Surveys. London: HM Stationery Office, 1995: In press

30 Stellman SD, Garfinkel L. Lung cancer risk is proportional to cigarette yield: evidence from a prospective study. *Prev Med* 1989; **18**: 518–25

31 Kaufman DIV, Palmer JC, Rosenberg L, Stolley P, Warshauer E, Shapiro S. Tar content of cigarettes in relation to lung cancer. *Am J Epidemiol* 1989; **129**: 703–11

32 International Agency for Research on Cancer. *Tobacco smoking.* Monograph 38. Lyon: IARC, 1986

33 Wald N, Baron J. *Smoking and Hormone-Related Disorders.* Oxford: Oxford University Press, 1990

34 Poswillo D, Alberman E. *Effects of Smoking on the Fetus, Neonate and Child.* Oxford: Oxford University Press, 1992

35 Parish S, Collins R, Peto R *et al.* Cigarette tar yield and non-fatal myocardial infarction: 14,000 UK cases and 32,000 controls. *BMJ* 1995; **311**: 471–7

36 Frost C, Fullerton FM, Stephen AM *et al.* The tar reduction study. Randomised trial of the effect of cigarette tar yield reduction on compensatory smoking. In press

37 Swann C, Froggatt P. The Research Programme of the Tobacco Products Research Trust, 1982–1995. In press

38 Department of Health. *Smoke-free for Health.* London: Department of Health, 1994

Tobacco and the developing world

Judith Mackay* and **John Crofton**†

*Asian Consultancy on Tobacco Control, Kowloon, Hong Kong; †University of Edinburgh, Edinburgh, UK

Tobacco consumption is increasing in developing countries, which will bear the brunt of the tobacco epidemic in the 21st century. If current smoking patterns continue, 7 of the world's 10 million annual deaths from tobacco in 2025 will occur in developing countries.

Compared with developed countries, more men and fewer women currently smoke in developing countries, but smoking among girls and women is increasing.

While indigenous tobacco production and consumption remain a major problem, of particular concern is the penetration by the transnational tobacco companies, bringing with them denial of the health evidence, sophisticated advertising and promotion, threats of trade sanctions based on tobacco trade, and opposition to tobacco control measures, in particular promotional bans and tobacco tax policy.

Developing countries must urgently devise and implement national tobacco control policies, but many governments have little experience in the new non-communicable disease epidemic or in countering the transnational tobacco companies.

With the decrease in smoking prevalence in developed countries, the multinational tobacco companies are now moving massive resources to boosting sales in developing countries (see both Daynard and Pollock in this issue). In some developing countries, indigenous tobacco production and consumption present major problems. Many people and governments in these countries are not yet fully aware of the risks and lack the resources to counter ruthless marketing by the industry. If not prevented, there will be an appalling future increase in tobacco-related disease, disability and death[1].

History

Columbus brought information on smoking tobacco to Europe in 1492. The habit was later found to be extensive in South America[2]. In 1558, the tobacco plant itself reached Europe where pipe smoking spread rapidly. By 1525 tobacco trade had already been established between the

Caribbean and India, extending soon afterwards to China, Japan and the Malay peninsula[3,4]. About the same time, the Portuguese and Spanish brought tobacco down the east coast of Africa, and by 1560 it was being used in Central Africa[5] also. By the 17th century, tobacco was being produced in Russia, Persia, India and Japan[6].

The invention of the cigarette machine in the early 20th century created further interest in the large potential markets for tobacco in developing countries. On hearing of its invention, James B. Duke (1865–1925), the tycoon who established British American Tobacco (BAT), said: 'bring me the atlas'. He looked at the population figures and noted 'China: 430,000,000. That', he said, 'is where we are going to sell cigarettes' and 'that' was China[7].

By the beginning of this century, BAT was advertising throughout China[8]. By 1911, there were huge and widespread BAT posters[8] and even sponsored theatre performances[9]. By the 1920s, BAT awarded university scholarships in Hong Kong[10].

Chinese Government opposition, based on its own tobacco monopoly, was countered through action via the American and British governments[8]. Chinese annual consumption of cigarettes had risen from the negligible level of the 1890s to 100 billion cigarettes in the 1930s, a rise ascribed to the business practices of the cigarette industry[11]. When forced in 1952 to leave China, BAT forecast 'we will be back'—and so they are[12].

Following recognition of the lethal effects of tobacco, the potential threat to developing countries was dubbed, in an editorial in the *British Medical Journal* in 1971, as 'exporting tobacco slavery'[13].

The difficulties in countering the threat were recognised and addressed in the 1983 World Health Organization report *Smoking Control Strategies in Developing Countries*[14]; they were also emphasized in the 1983 report of the Royal College of Physicians of London[15]. Yet 2 years later, Brazil earned the dubious distinction of being the first developing country in which smoking was labelled by WHO as the leading cause of death[16].

In 1985, 73% of the world's tobacco was grown in developing countries[17], using land that could otherwise be used to grow food. Yet 63% of developing countries were spending more on importing tobacco than exporting it[18]. Although the epidemic lagged behind western countries, at a 1987 WHO Western Pacific Regional meeting on Tobacco or Health, it was emphasized that heart, circulatory disorders and cancer—all tobacco-related—were already the most common causes of death in Asia. Tobacco was causing developing countries twin problems—health and economic—that persist to this day.

During the last decade, as markets began to decline in developed countries, the transnational companies have been looking even harder towards developing countries. Glowing accounts of successful tobacco marketing in Asia, and the future potential there, have been given by the major companies: Philip Morris[19], British American Tobacco (BAT) and Rothmans (annual reports).

One tobacco industry executive summed it up succinctly: 'you know what we want? We want Asia'[20]. It would hardly matter whether all smokers in a country with a small population like Britain stopped smoking tomorrow, if the tobacco companies could capture the massive third world markets.

Review of present situation

Basic epidemiological information is lacking in many developing countries, some of which have still not undertaken a national survey on smoking prevalence. Of those that have, few reliable or country-wide surveys were done earlier than 10 years ago, so that information on trends is scanty.

In general, patterns of smoking are different in developing and developed countries: more men (50–60%) but fewer women (2–10%) smoke in developing countries compared with developed countries, where approximately 25–30% of both men and women smoke[21]. But, as in developed countries, smoking starts among young people and for much the same reasons[22].

Girls start smoking later than boys and smoke fewer cigarettes; smoking has been considered socially unacceptable for women (with exceptions, such as certain areas of India, Nepal, Papua New Guinea, northern Thailand, and for Maoris); there may be religious constraints, for example in Muslim countries; women have had less spending power than men to buy cigarettes; rural women adhere to traditional methods of smoking, e.g. hubble-bubble pipes, and are therefore exposed to a lower dosage of tobacco; and in some areas, such as parts of India and the Middle East, women use tobacco in other forms, such as chewing tobacco (see Pershagen in this issue). There may be significant under-reporting of smoking among women in countries where it is culturally less acceptable for women to smoke.

Because of poverty in Africa, many smokers can only afford a few cigarettes per day (see Amos in this issue). Even in Asia, smokers smoke on average fewer cigarettes than in western countries. For example, smokers in China smoke on average 11–15 cigarettes daily.

In Africa, more girls and women are taking up the habit[23]. In many areas of India, while only 3% of women smoke manufactured cigarettes, 50–60% chew tobacco[21]. In South America, while cigarette smoking is lower among women (20%) than among men (37%), there is a wide variation in prevalence of smoking among women, from 3% in La Paz,

Bolivia to 49% in Buenos Aires, Argentina[3]. In the eastern Mediterranean, approximately 40–50% of men smoke, but smoking by eastern Mediterranean women is often considered to be vulgar and improper, even immoral. Female smoking is still low but increasing in professionals in the Middle East and North African region (Sherif Omar, personal communication).

Future trends

Between 1986 and 1991, world per capita consumption decreased by less than 1%. The Food and Agriculture Organisation of the United Nations estimates that between the years 1984–86 and 2000 tobacco consumption in developed countries will decrease by 11% but in developing countries it will increase by 10%. Of total world consumption in 1974–76, 49% was in developing countries. This rose to 61% in 1984–86 and is estimated to rise to 71% by the year 2000[24].

Between 1986 and 1991, per capita consumption declined in Africa by 11%, in North America by 13%, in South America by 7% and in the European Community by 3.5%. Only in Eastern Europe and Asia did per capita consumption increase, by 2% and 13.5%, respectively. Asia already accounts for about half the world cigarette consumption and this share is increasing at a much greater rate than the total world growth. The transnational companies have estimated that the market for cigarettes in Asia will grow by 33% between 1991 and the year 2000. This is compared with the predicted global increase of 5.2% in volume and 4.4% in monetary value (although, excluding China, global sales would actually fall in volume)[25].

The numbers of smokers will increase for several reasons: (i) increase in population in the Third World, from 4.5 billion to 7.1 billion by 2025[26,27]; (ii) increase in smoking prevalence, especially in the young, and especially in towns, initially in the better educated, and as a result of increasing affluence[3,28]; (iii) a likely increase in smoking among women, owing to intensive tobacco marketing and to decrease in the social taboo for women; (iv) ignorance of the health risks, particularly among the rural and uneducated, but even among health professionals[29]; (v) the lack of funding for control measures and the difficulty in implementing these, especially in rural areas; and (vi) above all, the intensive and ruthless marketing by multinational tobacco companies.

Not all these factors apply to all developing countries, but most apply to most. This likely explosion of tobacco consumption, unless prevented, will result in not only a human but also an economic burden of medical and health costs, lost productivity, loss of the use of land that could be used to grow nutritious food, loss of foreign exchange if cigarettes are imported, environmental costs including costs of fires, use of wood to cure tobacco, smokers' litter, as well as the costs to the individual smoker and his/her family.

On present trends worldwide, annual deaths from cigarettes are expected to rise from the current 3 million to about 10 million by 2025, and 7 million of these deaths will be in developing countries. Two million will be in China alone[1].

National action

Background

Developing countries are at very different stages in the development of the tobacco epidemic and in actions to counter that epidemic. If a country has yet taken little action the first essential is to recruit medical interest in the problem. This can be done via visiting foreign consultants. Oncologists, cardiologists or respiratory physicians, invited for their general expertise, can strongly emphasize the importance of smoking and help to create a responsible medical climate locally.

A similar influence can derive from international meetings of the relevant specialty where smoking problems are given a significant place. Once interested, the doctors, with their prestige and social standing, can then influence opinion and decision makers in their country to take up the problem.

WHO and international non-governmental organisations (NGOs) may then be able to help: WHO working through government contacts, NGOs through their national affiliated body or bodies and professional groups. Dr H. Mahler, a previous Director General of WHO, called this 'the pincer movement'.

National tobacco control policy

The key to tobacco control lies in prevention. The essential elements of a national tobacco control policy are the same for all countries.

Data collection Conclusive world data on the hazards of tobacco already exist on which developing countries can base preventive public health action now, without waiting for any further research.

However, surveys on tobacco prevalence; mortality and morbidity related to tobacco use; attitudinal surveys; the economic impact of tobacco; and evaluation of tobacco control measures remain important. Such national data are useful in order to convince opinion leaders, politicians and the general public of the importance both of the problem and of the urgent necessity to address it. While many developing countries have not yet done a national prevalence survey, even fewer have even partially evaluated the cost of tobacco to their economy. Data are particularly lacking for Africa.

In September 1995, WHO held a meeting on global standardised guidelines for studies, including core questions, for simple studies for developing countries which are:

If only 1 question can be asked:
1. Do you now smoke daily, occasionally or not at all?

If 2 questions can be asked:
1 above and a 2nd Q on EITHER on daily consumption OR on previous history:
1. (above)
and
2a. How many of the following items do you smoke, chew or apply each day?
      . . . . . . manufactured cigarettes
      . . . . . hand-rolled cigarettes
      . . . . . bidis
      . . . . . pipefuls of tobacco
      . . . . . betel quids
      . . . . . snuff
OR:
2b. Have you ever smoked daily, occasionally, or not at all?
      . . . . . . daily
      . . . . . . occasionally
      . . . . . . not at all or less than 100 cigarettes in your lifetime

If more questions can be asked:
1. Have you ever smoked? (Y/N). If yes, go to next question.
2. Have ever smoked at least 100 cigarettes or the equivalent amount of tobacco in your lifetime? (Y/N)
3. Have you ever smoked daily? (Y/N)
4. Do you now smoke daily, occasionally, or not at all?
     (D, O, Not at all)
5. On average, what number of the following items do/did you smoke per day?
      . . . . . . manufactured cigarettes
      . . . . . hand-rolled cigarettes
      . . . . . bidis
      . . . . . pipefuls of tobacco
      . . . . . cigares/cheroots/cigarillos
      . . . . . goza/hookah

6. How many years have you smoked/did you smoke daily?
7. For ex-smokers: How long has it been since you last smoked?
   — less than one month
   — one month or longer but less than six months
   — six months or longer but less than one year
   — one year or longer but less than five years
   — five years or longer but less than ten years
   — 10 years or longer

Establishment of a national tobacco control policy programme and national coordinating organization WHO has recommended the establishment of a national focal point to stimulate, support and coordinate all anti-tobacco activities. Many developing countries have established such organizations over the last decade, either within Ministries of Health or by non-governmental organizations (NGOs). World experience has shown the vital importance of government commitment, funding and action in establishing a national programme to reduce the tobacco epidemic.

Health information and education The enormous difference in funding available for health education in comparison to the money spent on promotion by the tobacco companies remains an unsolved problem in all developing countries. In contrast to the attractive images used by the tobacco companies, many health educators have used depressing, even boring health statistics and finger-wagging 'don't smoke' messages which may encourage adults to quit, but seem to have little effect in preventing young people from starting smoking. But it is still not known whether this more authoritative approach works better in countries where teaching is more traditional and teachers are respected by students. Health education in developing countries, especially that geared for youth, is now beginning to move towards positive, healthy lifestyle images, and teaching young people how to say no.

Health education is expanding. In 1993, 31 out of the 35 countries in the WHO Western Pacific Region celebrated World No Tobacco Day on 31 May.

Legislation Legislation also has an important role to play. Its desirable components are now well recognised (see Reid in this issue). We comment below on individual items from the point of view of developing countries. Legislation will only be enacted after appropriate build up of national opinion, especially among decision makers. If the law is to be effective, it is essential that a government department be made responsible for monitoring its implementation and prosecuting for breaches of the law. Penalties for breach must be sufficiently substantial to deter even very rich multinational companies, e.g. very high fines, banning that company's imports for a specific number of months. A combined approach of health education and legislation, such as in Singapore and Hong Kong, is particularly effective.

1. **Ban on tobacco promotion.** Studies have shown that children are aware of and are influenced by tobacco advertising[30,31]. By 1991, 27 countries had total bans on advertising, 12 had strong partial bans, and many countries had moderate partial bans[32]. Partial bans have only partial effects, and even developing countries with comprehensive bans find these are frequently circumvented by ingenious indirect advertising and sponsorship. This includes sponsorship of sports, arts, TV and radio programmes, medical establishments and pop concerts; 'infomercials' (adverts that are dressed up as public affairs shows, as broadcast on television in China); product placement in films (e.g. Hong Kong) and other goods (virtually all countries) abound. Dealing with this is one of the major problems for developing countries. Satellite broadcasting is only one particular problem.

2. **Discouraging smoking among youth.** Few developing countries ban sales to minors, probably because of the difficulties envisaged in enforcing the law. This is the one and only tobacco control law supported by the tobacco industry in developing countries, a sure indication of its ineffectiveness.

3. **Effective, rotating health warnings.** By 1991, 70 countries worldwide required health warnings on cigarette packets[32]. With few exceptions, such as Thailand, health warnings in developing countries (for those that have any) are single and feeble.

4. **Limits on harmful substances.** Lowering the very high tar levels (e.g. average over 30 mg) found in cigarettes in developing countries can prevent about one third of lung cancer. A ceiling of about 10–15 mg of tar per cigarette is recommended[33], below which smokers compensate by smoking more cigarettes, drawing more often on each cigarette, inhaling more deeply and smoking further down each butt. Smokers have an exaggerated perception of the benefits of low tar cigarettes, so the tobacco companies should never be allowed to suggest that a lower tar cigarette is a 'safe' cigarette. The goal should always be to quit. An appropriate warning system would be to label cigarette categories as 'Dangerous', 'Very dangerous' and 'Most dangerous', or a visual warning, such as the picture of a skull and crossbones.

5. **Smokeless tobacco** (see Pershagen in this issue). In India, where chewing tobacco is a long-established custom, community programmes have been successful in reducing chewing tobacco among rural women[34,35]. New forms of manufactured tobacco products are

constantly being launched, such as chewing and sucking tobacco, and tobacco sweets[36,37]. Several developing countries in the Western Pacific region, where chewing tobacco has never been a popular habit, have taken the opportunity to ban smokeless tobacco before it became established on their markets.

6. **Creation of smoke-free areas.** As it is now known that tobacco smoke is not only unpleasant to non-smokers but may also cause them to develop cancer[38], many developing countries have banned smoking in public areas, public transport and places of work, especially in health premises, schools and government offices. Two thirds of all adults and virtually all young children in developing countries are non-smokers; thus the freedom of the majority to breathe clean air is a more vital consideration than the freedom of smokers to smoke in public places. Virtually all flights within Asia are now smoke-free, as are some long-haul flights from Asia.

Tobacco price and taxation policy Progressive increase of tax on cigarettes above the rates of increase for inflation and for disposable income is a very effective way of both discouraging smoking and also increasing government revenue (see Townsend in this issue). Smokers polled in developing countries give cost and health as their two main reasons for quitting. Increasing tax has a particularly beneficial effect upon young people and the poor, who have less money to spend, and are therefore more likely to quit. While in the USA, for example, for every 10% tax increase there is a 4% decrease in smokers[39], and a 14% decrease in teenage smokers[40], a study from Papua New Guinea suggests that this resulting decrease in smoking may be even greater in developing countries[41]. WHO has noted that 'millions of lives could be saved if steep taxes were imposed on tobacco'[42]. Care needs to be exercised in increasing taxes so that these are not seen as punitive or 'anti-smoker', and also that it does not place too harsh a burden on lower-income smokers who are unable to quit. Finance Ministers need to be reminded that they will gain, not lose, revenue by increasing tobacco tax (see Townsend in this issue).

Another method of utilising tobacco taxation as a means to improve health is to implement differential taxation on higher tar cigarettes.

Very few developing countries have earmarked any percentage of tobacco tax revenue to fund anti-tobacco activities. An exception is Peru, where a percentage of tobacco tax is used for anti-cancer activities, research and treatment.

Litigation Although successful litigation based on the harmfulness of both active and passive smoking has been undertaken in developed countries, there has not yet been a successful case brought against the tobacco industry or an employer in any developing country (see Howard in this issue). Where there are state tobacco monopolies, suing the tobacco industry would involve the unlikely situation of an individual suing the government of that country. It would also require funding and expertise far beyond the means of many individuals or health societies in developing countries. Nevertheless, rulings in developed countries have been used in developing countries. For example, information on successful court cases based on passive smoking in the workplace can encourage employers in other countries to take action to provide a safe, smoke-free work environment.

International strategies relevant to developing countries

Role of international and regional health agencies

World Health Organization (WHO)   The WHO Representative and office may be the only long-term major international health organization permanently present in a developing country. WHO has effective access to the Ministries of Health and WHO policy statements are powerful: the knowledge that a suggested item of tobacco control legislation is a WHO recommendation can carry great weight in developing countries. WHO can also provide some funding for country projects, including research, meetings, seminars and visits by experts. The 1983 WHO Report *Smoking Control Strategies in Developing Countries*[14] remains a very useful guide.

The Western Pacific Regional Office of WHO has been particularly active in tobacco control, convening three working groups to advise on the problem, and producing two 5-year Action Plans (1990–1994 and 1995–1999). The latter calls for all governments (and all countries in the region except Australia, Japan and New Zealand are developing countries) to implement comprehensive tobacco control measures by 1999. These include a national policy and central coordinating agency on tobacco or health, health education, comprehensive tobacco control legislation and pricing policy. Highlights include:

- A call for a 'Tobacco advertising-free Region by the Year 2000' as part of comprehensive legislation on tobacco or health.
- The recommendation that a percentage of tobacco tax should be used to fund sports, arts and health promotion, so that sports and arts organisations do not suffer from the ban on tobacco sponsorship.

- Introduction of health information and advocacy on tobacco or health into medical curricula.
- Compliance with the International Civil Aviation Organization resolution that all airlines become smoke-free by 1996.
- Involvement of religious and other community groups in tobacco or health activities.
- The goal, for countries and areas with a long history of tobacco or health action, to decrease their tobacco consumption by at least 1–2% per annum.
- The goal, for countries and areas that had not previously taken significant action on tobacco or health to implement national action (with a view to reducing consumption during the next 2000–2004 Action Plan on Tobacco or Health).
- The goal, for all countries and areas, to prevent a rise in smoking among women.

Some developing countries have shown that tobacco control measures are not the prerogative of western nations; they can be implemented in developing nations; they can be implemented quickly; and they can be effective. For example, Singapore and Thailand in the Asia-Pacific region, and Botswana in Africa, have implemented comprehensive tobacco control measures.

International/regional non-governmental organizations (NGOs) International organizations like the International Union Against Cancer (UICC), the International Union Against Tuberculosis and Lung Disease (IUATLD) or Consumers International (CI) can encourage their member organizations in developing countries to take a public and political stand on the tobacco epidemic, and also can fund projects, research, meetings and the visits of experts.

Regional organizations are particularly useful, such as the Latin American Coordinating Committee on Smoking Control (LACCSC), or the Asia Pacific Association for the Control of Tobacco (APACT). Both these organizations hold annual regional meetings. Delegates, especially from the poorer countries, find the smaller regional meetings more supportive than the large, international conferences. Following the first 'All-Africa Tobacco Control Conference' in 1993, a Tobacco Control Commission of Africa was formed in 1994, to coordinate regional efforts and implement the recommendations of the 1993 conference (Dr Yussuf Saloojee, personal communication).

Representatives of the 6 different developing regions of the world met in special sessions at the 9th World Conference on Tobacco or Health in 1994 to discuss regional developments and plan future strategy.

Trans-national issues and strategies

Trans-national strategies   It is imperative that the health organisations, develop trans-national strategies, including those countering tobacco industry strategies, as the tobacco industry already has developed global, regional and national strategies (see articles by Chapman, by Pollock and by Daynard in this issue), which include:

- Denial of the health evidence.
- Promotion (see below).
- Attempts to prevent national governments taking tobacco control measures.
- Aggressive trade policies in association with US trade representatives, US Embassies, Consulates, and politicians.
- Strategies for 'dealing with anti-tobacco pressure groups'.
- Strategies for handling litigation.

Global aspects of promotion
- Satellite television promotion, especially sports sponsorship, cigarette 'holidays', on Internet etc.
- Overlap of broadcasting and tobacco advertising to neighbouring countries.
- Tobacco product placement in TV and cinema films, either produced in one country but shown throughout the world, or (already confirmed) in films made in developing countries.
- Coordinated circumvention of the spirit of promotion bans.

Smuggling   In 1992, the export of 171 billion cigarettes was recorded that were not accounted for in any recorded, legitimate imports. Between 10–35% of the world's cigarettes in international trade are smuggled[43]. Transborder smuggling is a global problem of advantage to the cigarette companies:

- It softens a market ahead of penetration.
- It circumvents any volume restrictions on imports (e.g. in China prior to 1995).
- The transnational tobacco companies still sell the cigarettes, so they do not lose financially (unlike the government, which loses tax).
- The transnational tobacco companies can use the smuggling argument to persuade governments not to raise cigarette taxes.
- It occurs especially across borders where there are large differentials in prices. In developing regions, the major problem lies between China and Hong Kong, but occurs in many other areas. To counter smuggling, countries can insist on package health warnings in the

local language (as in Thailand) or a stamp on each package to indicate that tax has been paid.

Agriculture and production   Most tobacco is smoked in the country of origin, but the remainder constitutes inter-country tobacco trade[18]. The western tobacco industry has begun switching farming and production to developing countries where there are cheaper labour costs.

Suggested global actions

1. An International Convention or Code on Tobacco or Health, similar to other international conventions such as those of the International Labour Organisation (ILO), is needed. This is especially important since global legislation, e.g. advertising regulations or laws, does not exist. UN resolutions on tobacco would be the appropriate first step in this process.
2. All UN agencies should produce recommendations, including tobacco in Children's Charters, Bills of Rights, International Civil Aviation Organization (ICAO), Food and Agriculture Organization (FAO) and World Bank resolutions and recommendations, etc., where these have not already been issued and, specifically, that FAO and the World Bank should give assistance with alternative crops.
3. Model tobacco control recommendations (UICC[33]) and draft legislation (WHO) should be issued and re-issued, as a template for action by national governments. Model country examples, like Singapore, should be circulated to other countries.
4. Developing countries should have ready access to global sources of information, e.g. those from WHO, UICC, Globalink, IATH, 'Tobacco Control', etc. (see below).
5. An International Coalition of Non-Governmental Organizations for Tobacco Control was established at the 9th World Conference on Tobacco or Health in 1994. Members include the International Union Against Tuberculosis and Lung Disease (IUATLD), the International Union for Health Promotion and Education (IUHPE), the International Union Against Cancer (UICC), International Doctors Against Tobacco (IDAT), Consumers International (CI), the International Society and Federation of Cardiology (ISFC), the International Agency on Tobacco and Health (IATH), the International Network of Women Against Tobacco (INWAT) and others. The aim is to present a cohesive and common front on specific issues and to avoid duplication of effort.
6. Each international NGO should, in addition to encouraging action by their member organisations, agree upon a specific task. For instance,

UICC has addressed national tobacco-control policy and the IUATLD has researched and issued guidelines for incorporating tobacco into medical school curricula.

7. WHO and various NGOs should cooperate at international, regional and national level; for example, a regional conference or workshop could derive greater strength from the input of several organizations.

8. There should be a Plenary Session on tobacco in every conference organised by relevant NGOs, as well as these meetings being decreed 'smoke-free meetings'.

9. Other NGO agencies need to be mobilised, for example, youth, women's, environmental, religious and other community groups.

10. International networks of lawyers, doctors and others, including members from developing countries, should be established. Three international organisations, International Network of Women against Tobacco, Doctors against Tobacco, and Dentists against Tobacco have recently been initiated.

11. Information links, including electronic links, should be strengthened and developed, such as Globalink and the International Agency on Tobacco or Health.

Relevant sources of information

The following may be found useful by those working in developing countries:

1. Your local WHO Representative: you could trace this source through your Ministry of Health.

2. Your Regional WHO Office.

3. The WHO Tobacco or Health Unit, Geneva. (Director, WHO Programme on Tobacco or Health, Programme on Substance Abuse, World Health Organization, 1211 Geneva 27, Switzerland. Tel: 41-22-791-3493, Fax: 41-22-791-4851).

4. The International Union Against Cancer (UICC). (Head, Education Department, International Union Against Cancer, Rue du Conseil-General 3, 1205 Geneva, Switzerland. Tel: 41-22-320-1811, Fax: 41-22-320-1810).

5. Globalink, centralised at UICC. (Globalink System Manager, UICC, Rue du Conseil-General 3, 1205 Geneva, Switzerland. Tel: 41-22-320-1811, Fax: 41-22-320-1810). Globalink is the International Computer Network of the International Union Against Cancer, that can be accessed with a personal computer, a modem and a standard telephone line from anywhere in the world. It provides e-mail, news

bulletins, electronic conferences and several databases. Hard copies of regional monthly news bulletins are available in some regions for those without electronic access.

6. The International Union Against Tuberculosis and Lung Disease (IUATLD). (Executive Director, International Union Against Tuberculosis and Lung Disease, 68 Boulevard Saint-Michel, 75006 Paris, France. Tel: 33-1-46.33.08.30, Fax: 33-1-43.29.90.87).

7. International Agency on Tobacco and Health (IATH). (Director, International Agency on Tobacco and Health, c/o ASH, 109 Gloucester Place, London W1H 3PH,UK. Tel: 44-171-935-3519, Fax: 44-171-935-3463).

References

1 Peto R, Lopez AD, Boreham J, Thun M, Heath Jr C. *Mortality from smoking in developed countries 1950–2000*. Oxford: Oxford University Press, 1994: pp 101–3

2 *Encyclopaedia Britannica*, 9th edn. 1888; **XXIII**: 423–7

3 US Department of Health and Human Services. *Smoking and Health in the Americas*. A 1992 report of the Surgeon General, in collaboration with the Pan American Health Organization. Atlanta, Georgia: US Department of Health and Human Services, Public Health Service, Centers for Disease Control, National Center for Chronic Disease Prevention and Health Promotion, Office on Smoking and Health, 1992, DHHS Publication No (CDC) 92-8419

4 Couling S. *The Encyclopaedia Sinica*. Hong Kong: Oxford University Press, 1917

5 IARC Monographs on the evaluation of the carcinogenic risk of chemicals to humans. Volume 38. *Tobacco Smoking*. Lyon, France: IARC, 1986: 48

6 Morton L. *Robert Carter of Nomini Hall. A Virginia tobacco planter of the eighteenth century*. 2nd edn. Princeton, New Jersey: Princeton University Press, 1945

7 Dobson RP. *China Cycle*. London: 1946: p 18

8 Cochran S. *Big Business in China: Sino-foreign Rivalry in the Cigarette Industry, 1890–1930*. Cambridge, Massachusetts and London, UK: Harvard University Press, 1980

9 Jansen W. *Chinese Economic Monthly* 1924 (11 August): 12

10 Ting Wen-chiang, ed. Free enterprise in China: the case of a cigarette concern, 1905–1953. *Pacific Historical Rev* 1960; **29** (4): 389n18

11 Tennant. Cigarette and tobacco trade in China. *Chinese Economic Bull* 1925; **225**: 338

12 *A British Success: A World Class Performance*. BAT Industries, London. Pamphlet to the Ordinary Shareholders. 21.8.89: p 12

13 Editorial. World action on smoking. *BMJ* 1971; **4**: 65–6

14 World Health Organization. *Smoking Control Strategies in Developing Countries*. WHO Technical Report Series No 695. Geneva: WHO, 1983

15 Royal College of Physicians of London. *Health or Smoking?* London: Pitman, 1983

16 Editorial. Brazil tops Third World league for deaths from smoking. *New Scientist* 1985; **105** (1443): 8

17 Food and Agriculture Organisation of the United Nations. *FAO Production Yearbook*, Vol.39. Rome: FAO, 1985: p 211

18 Chapman S, Wong WL. *Tobacco Control in the Third World: A Resource Atlas*. Penang, Malaysia: International Organization of Consumers Unions, 1990

19 Scull R. (Vice President, Philip Morris Asia.) Bright future predicted for Asia Pacific. *World Tobacco* 1986; **94**: 35–41

20 Interview with the Tobacco Reporter. Reported by Heise L. Unhealthy alliance. *World Watch* 1988; **1**: 22

21 Chollat-Traquet C. *Women and Tobacco*. Geneva: World Health Organization, 1992
22 *Smoking and Youth in China 1992. Review and Recommendations*. Geneva & London: International Union Against Cancer and Cancer Research Campaign, 1993
23 Granworth H, Stanley K, Lopez AD. *Time Trends in Mortality for Cancer*. WHO/CAN/88.5
24 The Food and Agriculture Organisation of the United Nations. *Tobacco Supply Demand and Trade Projections 1995 and 2000*. Rome: FAO, 1990
25 *Tobacco Markets in Asia*. London: Euromonitor, 1993
26 United Nations. *World Population Prospects 1990*. New York: United Nations, 1991: pp 226–31
27 United Nations. *Sex and Age Distributions of Population. The 1990 Revision*. New York: United Nations, 1991: p 4
28 Weng XZ, Zhou YC, Su AM. Random sampling survey of smoking prevalence in the middle school students of Beijing. *Proceedings of the Seventh World Conference on Tobacco and Health*, Perth, Western Australia, 1990: p 286
29 Weng XZ, Hong ZG, Chen DY. Smoking prevalence in Chinese aged 15 and above. Report of 1984 first national prevalence survey. *Chin Med J (Eng)* 1987; **100** (11): 886–92
30 Charlton A. Children's advertisement-awareness related to their views on smoking. *Health Educ J* 1986; **45**: 75–8
31 Chapman S. *Cigarette Advertising and Smoking—A Review of the Evidence*. London: British Medical Association, 1985: p 12
32 Roemer R. *Legislative Action to Combat the World Tobacco Epidemic*. 2nd edn. Geneva: World Health Organization, 1993
33 Gray N, Daube M. *Guidelines for Smoking Control*. 2nd edn. Geneva: International Union Against Cancer, 1980
34 Aghi M. Psychosocial aspects of acquisition and cessation of tobacco habits in India. *World Smoking and Health* Summer 1987: pp 4–7
35 Aghi MB. Strategy of oral cancer control among rural Indian women to meet the goal of Health for All by the Year 2000. Paper presented at *8th World Conference on Tobacco or Health*, Buenos Aires, Argentina; 30 March–3 April 1992
36 *Smokeless Tobacco Control*. Report of a WHO Study Group. Technical Report Series 773. Geneva: World Health Organization, 1988
37 US Department of Health and Human Services. *The Health Consequences of Using Smokeless Tobacco*. A report of the advisory committee to the US Surgeon General. Bethesda, MD: US DHSS, 1986. NIH Publication No. 86-2874
38 Wald NJ, Nanchahal K, Thomson SG, Cuckle HS. Does breathing other people's tobacco smoke cause lung cancer? *BMJ* 1986; **293**: 1217–22
39 Warner KE. Cigarette taxation; doing good by doing well. *J Public Health Policy* 1984; **5**: 312–19
40 Lewit EM, Coate D, Grossman M. The effects of government regulation on teenage smoking. *J Law Economics* 1981; **24**: 545–69
41 Chapman S, Richardson J. Tobacco excise and declining tobacco consumption: the case of Papua New Guinea. *Am J Public Health* 1990; **60**: 537–40
42 World tobacco tax could help save millions of lives. Geneva: World Health Organization. *Tobacco Alert* 1984; **2** (4): 1
43 Collishaw N. Is the tobacco epidemic being brought under control, or just moved around? An international perspective. Manila, Philippines: World Health Organization Western Pacific Regional Office Working Group on Tobacco or Health, 5–8 April 1994

Index

NEXT ISSUE   BRITISH MEDICAL BULLETIN   Volume 52   Number 2   April 1996

Euthanasia

Scientific Editors

Gordon R Dunstan and Peter Lachmann

UNIVERSITY OF WOLVERHAMPTON
LEARNING RESOURCES

£58.00

WITHDRAWN

WP 0463276 1